50 BEST SHORT HIKES

UTAH'S
NATIONAL
PARKS

2ND EDITION

To my wife, Elain, whose support and companionship on the trail,

and in life, bring added joy to the journey

50 Best Short Hikes: Utah's National Parks
2nd edition 2014, 3rd printing 2016

Copyright © 2014 by Greg Witt

Library of Congress Cataloging-in-Publication Data

Witt, Greg, 1952–
    50 best short hikes : Utah's national parks / Greg Witt. — 2nd edition.
        pages cm
    Original edition: 50 best short hikes in Utah's national parks / Ron Adkison.
Berkeley, CA : Wilderness Press, 2001.
    Includes bibliographical references and index.
    ISBN 978-0-89997-724-9 (alk. paper) — ISBN 0-89997-724-3
    (alk. paper) — ISBN 978-0-89997-725-6 (eISBN)
    1. Hiking—Utah—Guidebooks. 2. National parks and reserves—Utah—Guidebooks.
    3. Utah—Guidebooks. I. Adkison, Ron. 50 best short hikes in Utah's national parks. II. Title.
III. Title: Fifty best short hikes. IV. Title: Utah's national parks.
    GV199.42.U8W58 2014
    796.5109792—dc23
                        2014001232

Front-cover photos of Queens Garden and Golden Throne (inset): © Greg Witt
Back-cover photo of Delicate Arch: © Neal Herbert/National Park Service
Interior photos: Greg Witt except where noted
Maps and cover design: Scott McGrew
Text design: Annie Long
Editor: Amber Kaye Henderson
Proofreader: Ritchey Halphen
Indexer: Rich Carlson

Manufactured in the United States of America

Published by: 🐸 **WILDERNESS PRESS**
                An imprint of AdventureKEEN
                2204 First Avenue South, Suite 102
                Birmingham, AL 35233
                800-443-7227
                info@wildernesspress.com

Visit **wildernesspress.com** for a complete listing of our books and for ordering information.

Distributed by Publishers Group West

Safety Notice
Although Wilderness Press and the author have made every attempt to ensure that the information in this book is accurate at press time, they are not responsible for any loss, damage, injury, or inconvenience that may occur while using this book. You are responsible for your own safety and health while in the wilderness. The fact that a trail is described in this book does not mean that it will be safe for you. Always check local conditions, know your own limitations, and consult a map and compass.

50 BEST SHORT HIKES

UTAH'S
NATIONAL
PARKS

2ND EDITION

Greg Witt

 WILDERNESS PRESS . . . *on the trail since 1967*

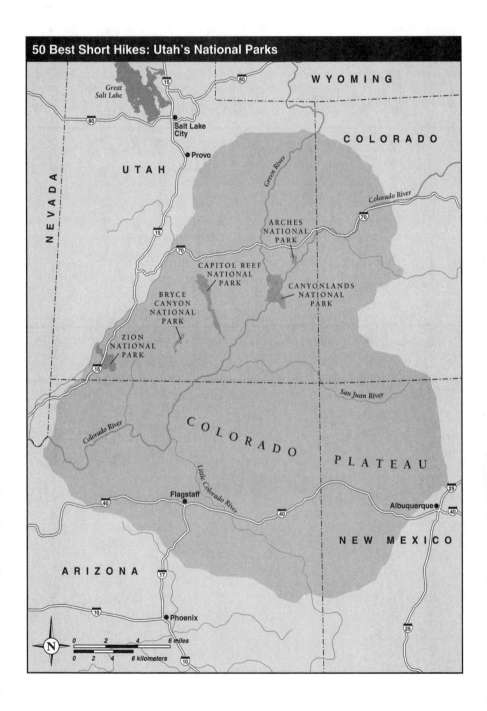

50 Best Short Hikes: Utah's National Parks

Contents

Acknowledgments

I'm fortunate to be in the business of connecting people with nature, both through my writing and by guiding hikers and trekkers on outdoor adventures—a wonderfully rewarding career with roots that can be traced to childhood. I have no recollection of what our living room furniture looked like in my boyhood home or what color carpet we had, or if we even *had* carpet. All of my memories center on experiences I had in the outdoors. I remember the pale-yellow Sears canvas tent and the smell of the khaki-green sleeping bags we used while camping in the Sierra Nevada. I remember the red asphalt of Zion's roads and driving through the Zion–Mt. Carmel tunnel in our 1955 Pontiac station wagon. I remember vividly our trips to Yellowstone, Crater Lake, and Glacier National Parks. I'm grateful for parents who planted the seeds of a love for the outdoors. So as I've written and researched the hikes in this book, I've also been reviving memories from 30, 40, and 50 years ago. What a thrill!

On these hikes I've shared the trail with dear friends, including Alan and Kris Colledge, Robert and Cathie Hooke (with whom we hiked five national parks in three days), and Nicki Preece. As always, my wife, Elain, has been close by with lively conversation on the trail as well as fresh ideas and thoughtful edits after the hike.

Every book is a collaborative effort, and the energetic assistance of Cami Lee in organizing photos and assembling maps is much appreciated. And once again it's been a pleasure working with the talented and professional folks at Menasha Ridge Press—Molly Merkle, Susan Haynes, Tim Jackson, Scott McGrew, Amber Kaye Henderson, and Ritchey Halphen—all of whom are relentlessly dedicated to delivering superbly readable and consistently valuable outdoor books.

—*Greg Witt*

The Very Best Short Hikes

Make the most of your national-park visit and discover the hikes that offer exactly what you're looking for. Here are my personal recommendations for the best of the best.

VERY BEST IN EACH NATIONAL PARK

9. **Devils Garden** *(Arches) More than a dozen arches in one hike, including Landscape Arch, the longest in the world*

15. **Queens Garden and Navajo Loop** *(Bryce Canyon) Venture below the rim into the heart of Bryce Canyon's hoodoos.*

27. **Elephant Hill to Chesler Park** *(Canyonlands) A slickrock trail with something for everyone—slots, washes, views, and varied terrain*

37. **Sulphur Creek** *(Capitol Reef) The creek is the trail as it flows through narrows and over waterfalls and ends up at the visitor center.*

44. **Angels Landing** *(Zion) Enter Refrigerator Canyon and ascend Walter's Wiggles before making the chain-assisted climb to the top of this spectacular canyon tower.*

VERY BEST VIEWS

1. **Park Avenue** *Walk down the Main Street of Arches National Park, flanked by immense fins and formations on both sides.*

23. **Crater View Trail and Upheaval Dome Overlook** *Gaze down into Upheaval Dome, with expansive views over the Canyonlands basin and beyond.*

24 **Grand View Point Trail** *An aptly named cliffside route overlooking the Canyonlands basin*

38. **Rim Overlook** *An easy walk from Sunset Point to Sunrise Point, two of Bryce's most popular viewpoints*

47. **Observation Point** *A splendid hike to a spectacular viewpoint above Zion Canyon*

VERY BEST WILDLIFE VIEWING

43. **Emerald Pools Trail** *Birds nest in the canyon's deep recesses, while wild turkeys and deer are frequently seen in the open areas of Zion Canyon.*

49. **Taylor Creek** *Songbirds, deer, and small mammals enjoy this shaded and wooded canyon as much as you will.*

VERY BEST ARCHAEOLOGY

21. **Aztec Butte Trail** *Beautifully preserved ancestral Puebloan granaries*
29. **Horseshoe Canyon** *Explore the Louvre of prehistoric rock art in the United States.*
39. **Capitol Gorge Trail to The Tanks** *Fremont Indian rock art and the Pioneer Register are etched on the canyon walls.*

VERY BEST FOR SMALL CHILDREN

3. **Windows Loop** *Kids can climb and play on three of the park's most impressive arches.*
4. **Double Arch** *A short walk to the second-largest arch in the park and a visual mind-bender*
22. **Whale Rock Trail** *High adventure in a short hike to the top of a slickrock dome*

VERY BEST FOR EASY STROLLING

2. **Balanced Rock** *A level loop around an immense gravity-defying rock*
14. **Rim Trail** *A level, paved path from Sunset Point to Sunrise Point, two of the park's favorite viewpoints*
20. **Mesa Arch Loop** *An easy walk to an arch perched on a cliff, with commanding views beyond*

VERY BEST ICONIC NATURAL FEATURES

5. **Delicate Arch** *The most iconic natural arch in the world*
13. **Peekaboo Loop** *Get up close and personal with the hoodoos from within the Bryce Amphitheater.*
30. **Hickman Bridge** *From the Fremont River trailhead, you'll walk to a natural bridge on a trail that passes underneath and through the opening.*
48. **Riverside Walk** *This easy stroll leads you into the mouth of the Zion Narrows.*

VERY BEST VEGETATION

11. **Bristlecone Loop** *A dense fir forest with bristlecone pines, some of Earth's oldest trees*
46. **Weeping Rock to Hidden Canyon** *Pass through various ecosystems, from cacti to ferns, all marked with interpretive signs.*

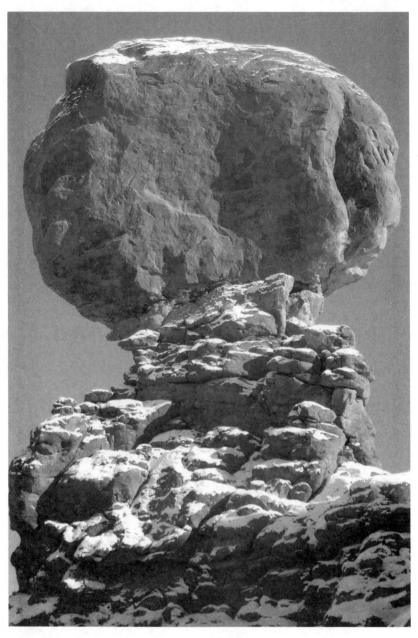

Balanced Rock in Arches National Park (see Hike 2, page 19)

INTRODUCTION

When was the last time you strapped on a pair of boots and let out a jaw-dropping "WOW"? If you can't remember, then it's been way too long.

But where are the guaranteed wow-producing hiking trails? Right here, in Utah's five national parks.

Within these pages you'll find trail descriptions and precise directions for dozens of the best day hikes in what I think is the most beautiful, fascinating, and diverse topography in the world—Arches, Bryce Canyon, Canyonlands, Capitol Reef, and Zion National Parks.

This book's title, *50 Best Short Hikes: Utah's National Parks,* has two operative words in the title: *best* and *short.* What you're about to uncover represents the very best of the thousands of miles of hiking trails within Utah's national parks. Many of these hikes are not only national treasures but are also rightly considered to be some of the best hikes in the world—Queens Garden, Delicate Arch, and Angels Landing certainly achieve that level of distinction. By *short* we mean day hikes of less than 8 miles, so enjoying two or even three of these hikes in a single day is doable.

This book was written as a trip-planning resource with families, casual hikers, and out-of-state visitors in mind, so that they can obtain maximum enjoyment from what might be a once-in-a-lifetime trip to Utah. Nevertheless, if you're an avid hiker and you live nearby, I can assure you that you'll still be amply rewarded by the hike descriptions and supplemental material provided herein.

Once you arrive at one of the parks, you'll want more than a drive-by experience. You'll be looking for family-friendly, easy-to-manage trails with bragging rights and photo ops included. All of these trails are hiker-tested, measured, and mapped.

Don't worry about running out of breathtaking scenery to explore. It will take you years to travel all these trails and unravel their mysteries. Petrified sand dunes, slot canyons, hoodoos (rock columns), and brilliant sandstone will fascinate you at every turn in the trail. Prairie dogs, prickly cacti, trickling springs, and star-studded skies will add even more to your adventure.

Each Utah national park has a distinct personality, profile, and palette. The more trails you try, the more you will understand why these areas are protected as national parks. Towering cliffs of brilliant orange, deep rust, mustard yellow, chocolate brown, creamy white, and muted green create an ever-shifting scenery above you and underfoot. The colors change even further with the help of clouds, rain, snow, or the setting sun.

In spite of their topographic differences, a single powerful force has shaped all five desert treasures: erosion. Eons of water, ice, and wind have created a kaleidoscope of geological features with Mother Nature's recipes. Each trail has been selected to help you see these geologic features up close.

I've tromped down every one of these trails, and dozens more, to identify the very best for you. Nature demands patience and curiosity to get the most from an outdoor experience. With *50 Best Short Hikes: Utah's National Parks*, you'll find what you're looking for—and so much more.

DRIVING IN THE NATIONAL PARKS

Most of the trailheads within this book, which are mainly front-country trails, are on paved and widely traveled roads in the more popular and widely accessed areas of the parks. But some trails in this book are found at the end of rocky, rutted, and occasionally impassable dirt roads. Some of these notably remote hikes include Tower Arch, Horseshoe Canyon, Elephant Hill, Golden Throne, Grand Wash, and Cable Mountain.

If your planned hike takes you to a trailhead on a dirt road, check first with the park's visitor center for current road conditions and a weather forecast. Recognize that even though a dirt road may be passable when you enter, conditions could change dramatically with rain or snow. Dirt roads in the desert could become muddy and slippery, and a flash flood could leave your return route washed out or strewn with rocks and debris.

If your trip involves one of the remote trailheads, always start the day with a full tank of gas and emergency provisions such as extra water, food, and clothing. Experienced desert travelers know that utility items in the trunk of the car, such as a shovel, towline, jack, and spare tire, can be lifesavers when your car is stuck or disabled.

HIKING SEASONS

Utah's five national parks are open year-round, though the availability of some services, such as shuttles, visitor centers, ranger-led programs, and campgrounds, will vary by season and from one park to another. Most of the hikes in this book are accessible and hikeable year-round. Even Bryce Canyon, with its high elevations and snowpack, can be enjoyed in winter on cross-country skis or snowshoes. In the arid desert of southern Utah, spring and fall often offer some of the most favorable hiking conditions. Regardless of when you plan to visit, it's important to plan carefully. National-park websites and visitor centers can provide planning information and weather forecasts, but your safety and enjoyment will depend on your own good judgment, preparation, and constant awareness.

PARK REGULATIONS

Visit **nps.gov** for additional rules.

- Campfires are prohibited except in front-country campgrounds, and wood gathering is not allowed.

- All vehicles, including mountain bikes, are restricted to designated vehicle routes; off-route travel is not permitted.

- Pets are not allowed on hiking trails.

- Hunting is prohibited.

- Do not use soap in or near water sources.

- Watch wildlife from a distance, and never feed wild animals.

- Swimming in potholes is not allowed unless the pothole is continually recharged by flowing water.

- The destruction, defacement, disturbance, or removal of natural or historical objects is prohibited.

USING THIS BOOK

When you think of Utah, theme parks don't generally come to mind. But Utah is home to five national parks—distinct parks with one common theme. That underlying and unifying theme is erosion. Each of Utah's national parks—Arches, Bryce Canyon, Canyonlands, Capitol Reef, and Zion—is a geologically themed wonderland where the subject is what happens to the earth's surface as a result of wind and water and time. Those results are the fantastic canyons, arches, hoodoos (rock columns), sandstone fins, and spires that decorate these parks.

Utah's national parks lie within a geographic region of the United States known as the Colorado Plateau, which spreads across 130,000 square miles of Utah, Arizona, New Mexico, and Colorado. It's an arid, high-elevation expanse that conspires against human settlement and showcases some of the most beautiful red-rock scenery and natural earth forms in the world. Ninety percent of the Colorado Plateau is drained by the Colorado River and its tributaries, and it has the highest concentration of National Park Service units in the country—10 national parks and 17 national monuments. Other national parks within the Colorado Plateau, though not in Utah, are the Grand Canyon, Mesa Verde, Black Canyon of the Gunnison, and Petrified Forest National Parks, as well as Chaco Culture National Historical Park.

To understand the geology of the Colorado Plateau, all you need to know are three basic steps:

◘ The area was thrust upward by forces within the earth.

◘ Tectonic plates collided, causing layers of earth to crinkle and tilt.

◘ Water cut and shaped the stone into canyons.

Simplified, yes, but everything you see in Utah's national parks indicates these three steps. And the desert climate, with its attendant lack of vegetation, makes the geology so much more visible and accessible. Think about it: If the Colorado Plateau were as forested as the Pacific Northwest, these national parks wouldn't exist because you would never notice the arches, hoodoos, slickrock, or magnificent sandstone monuments. So be thankful for the desert, which exposes this beautiful terrain and makes it so accessible for hikers.

As you visit Utah's national parks and immerse yourself in their wonders, you'll find new ways of looking at the land and uncover new ideas. Edward Abbey, that ever-quotable environmentalist of the Colorado Plateau, put it this way: "The land here is like a great book or a great symphony; it invites approaches toward comprehension on many levels, from all directions." Like Abbey, you'll find that each hike in this book offers something to learn, something new to ponder, or some riddle to answer. To enhance the learning and to make that knowledge accessible, I've included dozens of sidebars, photos, and interpretive aids—an added bonus, if you will—to bring the story of the land to life. These include information about the geology, history, flora, and fauna of the Colorado Plateau—facets that are common to all five national parks.

Utah's national parks lie within desert environments, which only make the life-forms more interesting as species—both plants and animals—adapt to the harsh climate. You'll find desert bighorn sheep that go most of the year without ever drinking water, bristlecone pines that live for thousands of years, or kangaroo rats that collect moisture with each outgoing breath. Deserts may look barren on the surface, but they are far from lifeless.

The parks featured here are open year-round, though some visitor centers and public facilities may be closed or have restricted hours during winter. Given their high elevation at or above 5,000 feet, the parks have great hiking during the peak summer season, even though other national parks in the desert Southwest will be scorchingly hot. Spring and fall are prime time for Utah's national parks and offer what most hikers consider ideal temperatures for hiking, along with long days, spring wildflowers, and lighter crowds. Winter can be magical as an occasional dusting of powder makes the red rock of Arches or Zion all the more photogenic. Bryce Canyon has groomed cross-country ski trails, and wildlife viewing in Zion is exceptional.

STAYING SAFE

Every route in this book is safe in the sense that it is a designated public trail within a national park. Most of the hikes in this book are considered front-country trails as opposed to remote backcountry trails, and as such the trails are well maintained, regularly patrolled and hiked by park rangers, and heavily used by visitors who come to Utah's national parks. Each year

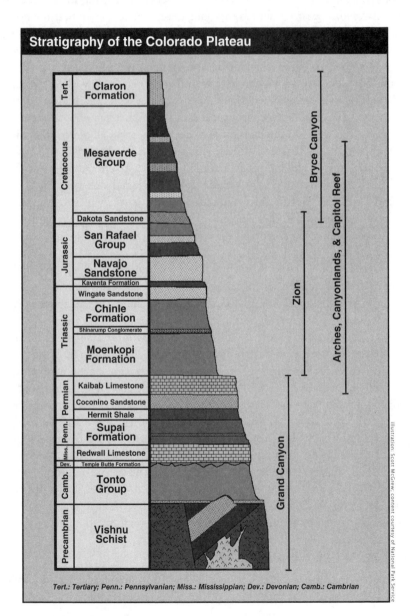

Illustration: Scott McGrew; content courtesy of National Park Service

millions of people find fun, rewarding, healthy, and life-transforming experiences while hiking in national parks.

However, the inherent risks and dangers in hiking in a national park or any outdoor setting are real. Rocks fall, rattlesnakes bite, flash floods roar down canyons, and the desert sun can toast you like a bagel. No ranger, guidebook, or trailhead sign can possibly protect you from every hazard. Nothing can take the place of personal responsibility, individual preparation, sound judgment, and constant awareness when hiking in the outdoors. With all that in mind, let's review some of the most common hazards you'll experience while hiking in Utah's national parks, along with the precautions and actions you should take in preparation for these hikes.

Even though most of these hikes are short, well known, well marked, and heavily used, you should be as mindful of precautions for these hikes as you would for any trail.

When visiting a national park, make the visitor center your first stop. Here you'll receive updated weather and trail notifications. Experienced rangers who know the trails can assist you in selecting the routes best suited to your experience and abilities.

The greatest risk factor for hikers on many of the trails in this book is the extremely hot and dry summer weather, with summer temperatures regularly in excess of 100°F. In the heat, be sure to wear a wide-brimmed hat and long sleeves. Carry water, wear sunglasses, apply sunscreen and lip balm liberally, and, when possible, plan your outings to avoid hiking in the heat of the midday sun.

Heat exhaustion, or hyperthermia, occurs when the body loses more fluid than it takes in. That can happen very quickly in the desert's high temperatures. Signs of heat exhaustion include nausea, vomiting, fatigue, headaches, pale appearance, stomach cramps, and cool clammy skin. If you or a member of your party experiences any of these signs, stop your hike immediately. Find a cool, shady area, and rest with your feet up. Drink fluids and eat something, while making a plan for returning to the trailhead or seeking assistance.

While hypothermia is usually associated with colder climes, it's a real risk here too, often due to the water in narrow canyons. Hypothermia occurs when the body cools to a dangerously low temperature. To prevent it, don't wear cotton clothing, and eat high-energy foods. Stop hiking if you observe uncontrollable shivering, poor coordination, fatigue, confusion, or slurred speech in any member of your party. Replace wet clothing with dry insulating layers, and plan to return to the trailhead or seek help.

Know where your sources of water are. For many of the hikes in this book, there is no water at the trailhead or on the trail, so plan ahead and fill your bottles at the visitor center or wherever reliable water supplies are found. Plan on drinking 1 gallon of water a day (or 1.5 gallons in the summer) while hiking.

You must always be mindful of trail conditions that can change over time and due to weather. Some of the easiest and most popular trails in Utah's national parks have been the site of fatalities due to extreme weather conditions (Zion's Riverside Walk is a notable example).

For all but the shortest hikes, bring along a lightweight backpack with plenty of water and something to snack on. Lack of adequate drinking water can sometimes be a critical issue on any of the hikes located in the arid desert climate of southern Utah.

It's best to avoid some of these unshaded hikes anytime the sun is high in the sky during the warmer months of the year. Walking will not be enjoyable at those times anyway.

Your backpack is a good receptacle for extra clothing as well. Because the high elevations and desert climate can experience wide swings in day and night temperatures, layering your attire is a good idea. In winter, take along two or more middleweight outer garments rather than relying on a single heavy or bulky jacket to keep you comfortable at all times.

Raingear, however, finds only occasional use in southern Utah. Usually, hikers have fair warning when a rainstorm is brewing—it's unusual for good weather to turn stormy within a short period of time. But always check the weather forecast.

Flash floods are rare, but they are still a risk that needs to be taken into account. Flash floods occur when rainfall, often miles away, falls onto slickrock or other nonabsorbent surfaces over a large drainage area and funnels into washes and channels. As channels constrict, the force of the floodwaters increases dramatically and carries debris and rocks. You can't outrun or swim in a flash flood. Avoid narrow canyons in rainstorms, and seek high ground.

You can take a mobile phone with you, but on most of these hikes you will not have cell service. Thus, as with all hiking, it's wise to let someone know where you are headed and when you expect to return.

Hikers on the more remote trails described in this book might want to bring along a flashlight (if there's any chance of being caught on the trail after dark); a map; a GPS unit, for fun as well as navigation; a whistle (for signaling); and a first-aid kit.

Rattlesnakes occasionally appear on the trails featured in this book. Typically, these creatures are as interested in avoiding contact with you

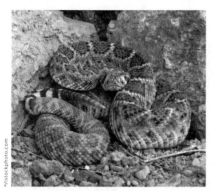
°/istockphoto.com

Western diamondback rattlesnake

as you are with them. But watch carefully where you put your feet, and especially your hands, during the warmer months, as you never want to startle a rattler. Most encounters between rattlesnakes and hikers occur in April and May, when snakes are out and about after a long hibernation period.

Insects are not as serious a problem in Utah's desert climate as they are in some other wilderness areas. But during the spring and summer, sand flies, deer flies, and midges can be occasional annoyances in some sandy washes and streambeds, so pack some insect repellent as a precaution. Tarantulas, scorpions, and black widow spiders are also present, but being bitten by one is a rare occurrence. For hikers, your best protection from being bitten is to stay on the trail and to keep your hands away from rocks or ledges where these creatures might be lurking.

Mountain lion encounters are extremely rare in Utah's national parks. Do, however, keep in mind that you must never run from any predatory animal, as this could trigger its chase instinct. Make yourself look large. Do not act fearful. Do anything you can to convince the animal that you are not its prey.

REDUCING YOUR IMPACT IN THE DESERT

Considering the significance of national parks to our nation's heritage, it's particularly important that you familiarize yourself with the Leave No Trace principles as you plan your visit to Utah's national parks. Visit lnt.org for more information. Follow the philosophy of "pack it in; pack it out." Here are a few additional pointers:

◘ Follow park regulations. Do not collect rocks, plants, or artifacts.

◘ Check the weather forecast, and plan your hike accordingly. Be prepared for emergencies.

◘ Deposit solid human waste in a hole 4–6 inches deep, at least 200 feet away from water, camps, and trails.

■ Do not approach or feed wildlife.

■ Yield to others on the trail. Step to the downhill side of the trail when encountering horses.

Additionally, in many parts of Utah's national parks, you'll encounter biological soil crusts (see page 18), which are an important part of the desert ecosystem. They prevent soil erosion, absorb and hold water, and provide nutrients to plants. But one footstep can destroy hundreds of years of growth. Please help protect these fragile crusts by learning to recognize them (you'll be instructed in the park's visitor information and on interpretive signage) and by walking on designated trails, bare rock, or streambeds.

Exciting experiences and vistas await, so now it's time to lace up your boots and hit the trail.

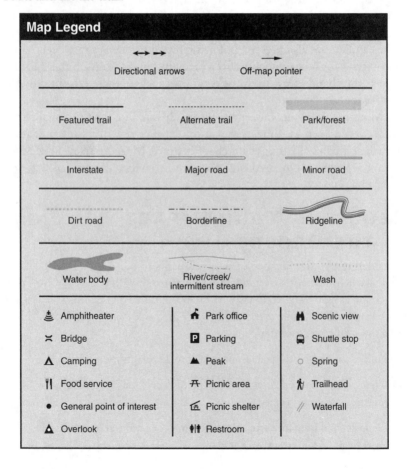

Map Legend

←→ →→ Directional arrows	→ Off-map pointer

Featured trail	Alternate trail	Park/forest

Interstate	Major road	Minor road

Dirt road	Borderline	Ridgeline

Water body	River/creek/ intermittent stream	Wash

♨ Amphitheater	♠ Park office	⌂ Scenic view
✄ Bridge	P Parking	🚌 Shuttle stop
A Camping	▲ Peak	○ Spring
⅋ Food service	♫ Picnic area	☀ Trailhead
• General point of interest	⌂ Picnic shelter	// Waterfall
△ Overlook	♦♦ Restroom	

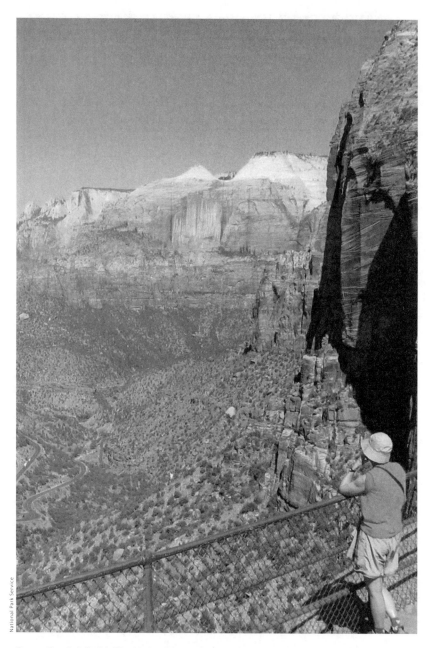

Canyon Overlook Trail in Zion National Park (see Hike 40, page 173)

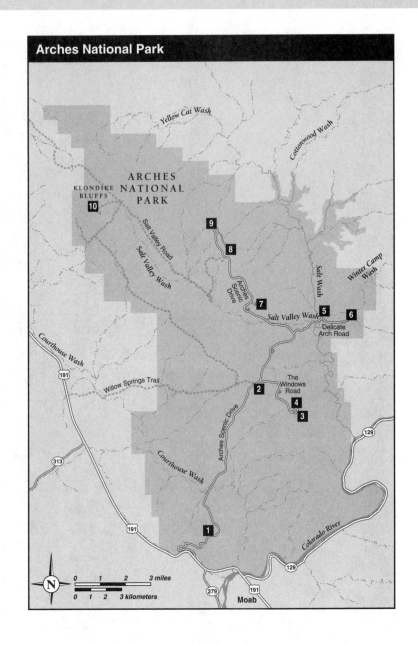

Arches National Park

ARCHES NATIONAL PARK

Park Overview

Arches National Park showcases the highest concentration of natural stone arches in the world—more than 2,400 of them. Along with the arches, you're treated to an amazing landscape of balanced rocks, soaring red-rock cliffs, monumental towers, and stately sandstone fins. It's inspiring scenery, with routes that are accessible to hikers of all ages and skill levels.

The arches and varied landforms spawn from an underground salt bed deposited 300 million years ago, when a sea flowed into the region and then evaporated. Subsequently, residue from floods, winds, and the ocean covered the salt bed and became compressed as rock, up to a mile thick in some places. Under this heavy rock layer, the salt bed shifted, liquefied, and buckled, causing domes to form and vertical cracks to appear in what we now see as fins.

Before being designated as a national monument in 1929 and a national park in 1971, the area had been inhabited for nearly 10,000 years, most recently by Fremont Indians and ancestral Puebloans, followed by Paiute and Ute tribes, Spanish missionaries, and Mormon pioneers.

JUST ONE DAY?

Arches is a compact park, ideally suited for visitors who want to take in the natural spectacle on short walks and hikes. Starting at the visitor center, continue into the park on what may be the most dramatic entrance to any national park in America as you ascend a road cut through sandstone to the Park Avenue Viewpoint. Continue on to Balanced Rock for a quick leg-stretcher, and then travel into the Windows section for a walk to the North and South Windows before heading up to Double Arch.

The must-do hike in Arches is Delicate Arch, the most iconic arch in Utah, if not the world. If you have any time and energy remaining, head to Devils Garden and pay a visit to Landscape Arch—quickly, before it collapses. This seemingly razor-thin span of rock continues to defy gravity and delight visitors.

◘ ◘ ◘

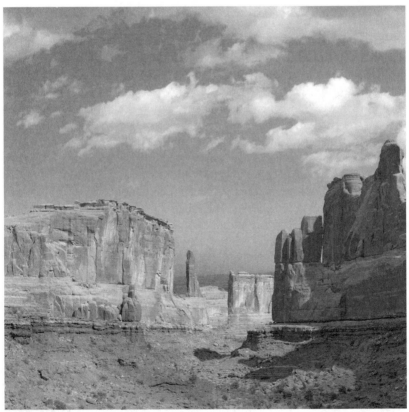

Park Avenue

1 Park Avenue

Trailhead Location: Park Avenue Viewpoint and parking area

Trail Use: Walking, hiking

Distance & Configuration: 2.0-mile out-and-back or 1.0-mile point-to-point with shuttle

Elevation Range: 4,550' at Park Avenue Viewpoint and Trailhead to 4,230' at Courthouse Towers Viewpoint

Facilities: None

Highlights: The perfect introductory hike in Arches National Park—a downhill walk along a canyon floor with towering walls and balanced rocks on both sides

DESCRIPTION

The Arches experience gets off to an impressive start as you leave the Arches Visitor Center and ascend a road carved below sandstone cliffs. Arriving at the Park Avenue Viewpoint and Trailhead, you'll need to decide whether to do this hike as a one-way—in which case you'll need a shuttle driver to meet you at the Courthouse Towers Viewpoint—or as a round-trip. If you have limited time and hope to pack as much hiking into your day as possible, do this as a one-way hike.

Park Avenue is a good introduction to desert hiking in general, where you'll discover sandy washes, slickrock, and immense sandstone cliffs. You'll encounter cacti and other desert plants and learn to recognize and avoid stepping on biological soil crusts. You'll learn to navigate by watching for cairns (small rock piles). The hike also exposes you to full sunlight, so you'll want to quickly establish the habit of packing water and staying hydrated. It's best to learn the ropes of desert hiking on a short and easy stretch such as Park Avenue, so you'll be prepared for bigger adventures deeper in the park. From observation points at either end of the trail, you'll be able to view most of the towers and walls of Park Avenue. But nothing can match the experience of hiking Park Avenue dwarfed by these monuments on all sides.

ROUTE

The observation deck at the trailhead captures a panorama not only of the canyon you're about to enter but also of the frequently snowcapped La Sal

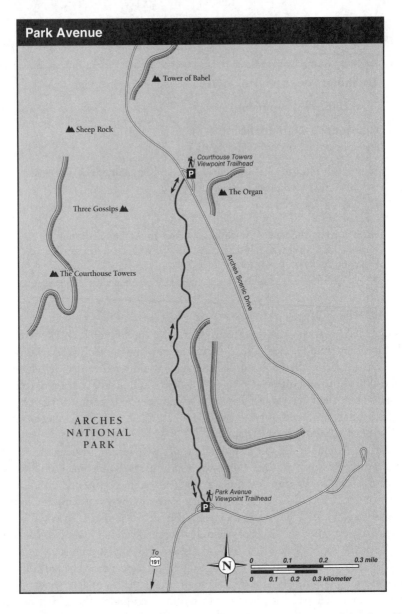

Park Avenue

Tower of Babel

Sheep Rock

Courthouse Towers
Viewpoint Trailhead

The Organ

Three Gossips

Arches Scenic Drive

The Courthouse Towers

ARCHES
NATIONAL
PARK

Park Avenue
Viewpoint Trailhead

To
191

N

| 0 | 0.1 | 0.2 | 0.3 mile |
| 0 | 0.1 | 0.2 | 0.3 kilometer |

Mountains, in the distance to the east. Walking down the paved sidewalk to the Park Avenue Viewpoint, you descend far enough into the canyon that the view and perspective of the Courthouse Towers and the canyon walls become even more dramatic.

From the observation deck, backtrack several paces; take the well-worn trail that veers left as it descends steeply into the canyon's wash. You will be on a slope dotted with Utah junipers and cacti. Continuing on, you'll find blackbrush, wavyleaf oak, Mormon tea, cliff rose, and single-leaf ash.

Once you reach the canyon floor, you'll be walking on dirt and sand on a bedrock layer of Navajo Sandstone. While the scenic beauty draws your eyes upward, you'll need to carefully watch your step, as potholed slickrock and sand can disguise parts of your route. To stay on the trail, watch for the occasional cairns, footprints, and a trail surface already compacted by other hikers.

To the north, an immense fin of Entrada Sandstone called the Tower of Babel rises 300 feet above the wash. There also, the Three Gossips—clustered pinnacles topped with head-shaped boulders—are so lifelike that you can almost hear them talking about you. Approaching the end of the wash, the trail ascends to meet the main park road. Cross Arches Scenic Drive at the crosswalk to the parking area and the Courthouse Towers Viewpoint, where you have fine views to the south of a 250-foot spire called The Organ.

Although there are no prominent arches along Park Avenue, you will notice several sandstone fins with deep erosion and fractures—arches in the making. From the Courthouse Towers Viewpoint, you'll spot a large pinnacle at the north end of the Sheep Rock fin to the northeast. This was

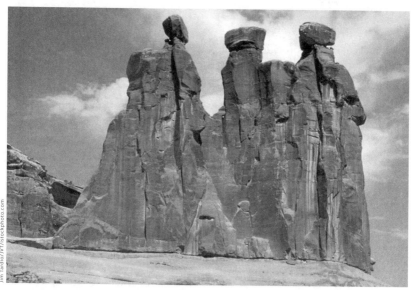

Jim Tardio/JVT/istockphoto.com

The Three Gossips

once the abutment of a now-collapsed arch, leading us to wonder what the park will look like 50, 5,000, or 50,000 years from today. What arches will collapse, and what new arches will form?

If you have a shuttle vehicle waiting for you at the Courthouse Towers Viewpoint, continue on into the heart of the park. Otherwise, retrace your route back to the Park Avenue Trailhead.

TO THE TRAILHEAD

GPS Coordinates: *Park Avenue Trailhead:* N38º 37.463' W109º 35.977' *Courthouse Towers Trailhead:* N38º 37.471' W109º 35.974'
From the Arches National Park entrance station, continue on Arches Entrance Road (the main park road) for 2.5 miles to the Park Avenue Viewpoint and parking area, on your left. If you plan to do this hike one-way, drive another 1.4 miles to Courthouse Towers Viewpoint, where you can leave a car in the lot on the right.

BIOLOGICAL SOIL CRUSTS: WATCH YOUR STEP

Biological soil crusts, also known as cryptobiotic soils, consist of cyanobacteria, lichens, and mosses. They act symbiotically as a kind of nursery for other desert organisms by binding loose soil particles to prevent erosion, providing nutrients to plants, and holding water. In high desert piñon-juniper and grassland ecosystems, biological soil crusts are the dominant nitrogen source. They cover nearly all desert soil 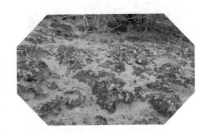 surfaces and are almost invisible in their early stages, but in maturity have a lumpish black appearance.

Please avoid walking on biological soils, as such pressure can do irreversible damage. Lichen recovery takes about 50 years, and moss recovery can take up to 250 years. You can protect these fragile soils by walking only on designated trails, bare rock, or streambeds.

2 Balanced Rock

Trailhead Location: Balanced Rock Parking Area

Trail Use: Walking, hiking

Distance & Configuration: 0.5-mile balloon

Elevation Range: 5,042' at trailhead to 5,070' at the loop's extension

Facilities: Vault toilet and picnic tables on Willow Flats Road, 0.2 mile north of trailhead

Highlights: A loop hike around one of the world's most-visited and widely photographed balanced rocks

DESCRIPTION

You'll see Balanced Rock in the distance and may even be tempted to drive right by as you head down the road in search of the more spectacular arches in the park. But this red-rock monolith is certainly worth a short stop, if for no other reason than to stretch your legs. In return you'll be rewarded with an up-close 360-degree view of this natural wonder that seems to defy gravity. The short walk gives you a chance to become familiar with the natural forces that created the arches farther down the road.

The general term *balanced rock* or *balancing rock* can be applied to any geologic formation in which a large boulder appears to be balancing on top of a pedestal or base. In reality, they are firmly attached to the pedestal (for example, the Entrada Sandstone's Dewey Bridge formation).

Balanced rocks are classified into different categories: glacial erratics, perched blocks, and erosional remnants. The balanced rock before you, along with the other balanced rocks and hoodoos throughout the Colorado Plateau, is clearly an erosional remnant, a formation of harder rock that remains after erosion has whittled away the softer material underneath in a process called differential erosion. In the process, the larger, more erosion-resistant layer on top now provides some protection to the softer layer on which it rests, thereby lengthening its precarious life.

While the centerpiece of this hike is Balanced Rock, don't let the views of the La Sal Mountains in the southeast go unnoticed. The La Sals are Utah's second-highest range, with its highest peak, Mount Peale, rising

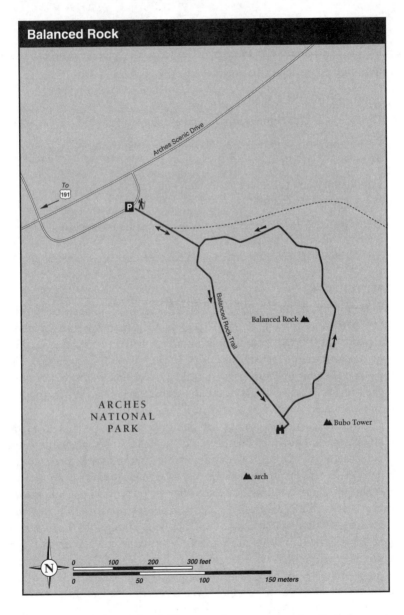

Balanced Rock

to 12,726 feet above sea level. The range's name, meaning "salt," was given by Spanish explorers, who may have doubted the existence of snowcapped desert peaks so far south. Instead, they believed the white summits were salt deposits, known to exist in the region.

ROUTE

From the parking area, the trail takes a direct route across desert brush to make a loop around Balanced Rock. The trail gently rises to a crest between Bubo Tower, a monolith fin and popular rock-climbing area to the immediate southeast of Balanced Rock. You've seen Balanced Rock from a mile or more in the distance and from the trailhead parking area, but there is simply no substitute for seeing it up close and making the full loop.

Standing below Balanced Rock presents a bit of an optical illusion, and it's difficult to really comprehend its size. Is it larger than a school bus? Smaller than a house? The top of Balanced Rock is about 128 feet above the base where you are standing, and the rock itself is about 55 feet above the pedestal on which it sits. The rock is roughly the size of three school buses.

From the trail you'll also see Elephant Butte to the southeast. Turret Arch and Double Arch, likely your next stop on your Arches visit, are visible to the right side of Elephant Butte, and the fanciful Parade of Elephants formation is south of Double Arch. If those views whet your appetite for some the park's most wondrous arches, then return to the parking area to continue your adventure.

TO THE TRAILHEAD

GPS Coordinates: N38° 42.104' W109° 33.958'

From the Arches National Park entrance station, continue on Arches Scenic Drive (the main park road) for 8.7 miles to the Balanced Rock Parking Area, on your left.

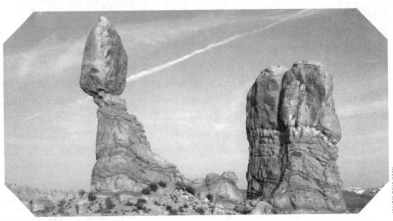

Balanced Rock

DO BALANCED ROCKS AND ARCHES FALL?

These fragile erosional remnants were gradually carved to their current form by wind, water, and other natural factors. Because balanced rocks and arches are constantly being eroded away, they don't last forever. Balanced Rock in Arches National Park once had a companion called Chip Off the Old Block, and it was also perfectly balanced until nature's forces caused it to fall in the winter of 1975–76.

Rockfall occurs frequently in Arches National Park and is most likely to happen after heavy rains or on winter afternoons as the sun quickly warms the cold rocks. During the night of August 8, 2008, Wall Arch, the 12th-largest arch in the park, collapsed. Arches and balanced rocks will eventually defy the forces holding them in place and succumb to gravity.

3 | Windows Loop

Trailhead Location: Windows Parking Area

Trail Use: Walking, hiking

Distance & Configuration: 1.0-mile loop

Elevation Range: 5,185' at trailhead to 5,325' within the arch

Facilities: Pit toilets at trailhead; no water

Highlights: An action-packed hike to three of the park's most impressive arches

DESCRIPTION

The Windows section of Arches National Park features a high concentration of many large and exceptionally photogenic arches. This short loop takes you past three favorites—North Window, South Window, and Turret Arch. The two Windows arches are part of the same sandstone fin, while Turret Arch is a separate castle-shaped fin with the turretlike tower rising on the south side of the fin.

When viewed together, the two windows take on the appearance of spectacles, and with not too much imagination the large bulbous rock between the two arches becomes the nose of some horrific monster.

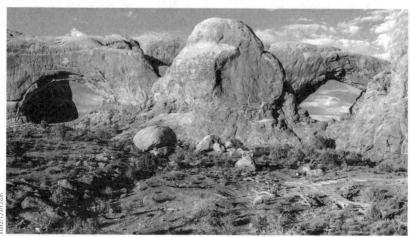

North and South Windows

Windows Loop

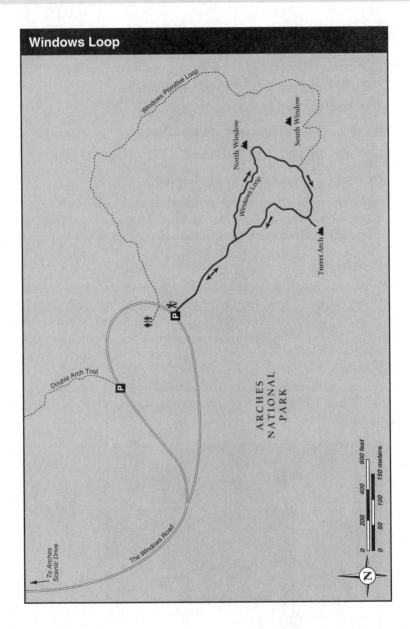

The immensity of these arches provides an inviting natural playground, and while the area beneath the North Window has been closed to public access, there is plenty of slickrock play area under the South Window and Turret Arch.

Unusual Turret Arch is one of a few arches that are significantly taller than they are wide. It takes a bit of scrambling to climb within the opening of the arch, but it's good fun and gives you access to some chutes and steep slickrock slopes to play on.

The Windows and Double Arch to the north share the same loop parking area, and because od their popularity, space in the large parking lot is often filled to overflowing. If you yearn to get off the beaten path, consider the primitive loop departing from the south end of the Windows Loop; it provides some solace, along with a particularly advantageous view of the North Window.

ROUTE

The wide and well-compacted route leads from the south side of the parking area across a flat stretch of blackbrush before arriving at a fork, with the Windows to the left and Turret Arch to the right. Taking the route to the left and tackling the trail in a clockwise direction leads up a stairway crafted in sandstone blocks in the direction of the Windows.

Arriving first at the larger North Window, you'll gaze through an arch that is 51 feet high and 93 feet wide. Because the base of the North Window sits almost level with the desert floor, it nicely frames a vista of distant mesas and cliffs to the southeast. Although direct access to the North Window has been closed to protect the surrounding landscape from damage, you'll still have fine views of the arch as you continue on toward the South Window. This section of trail also affords dramatic views of Turret Arch to the west.

A short spur leads up to the base of the South Window, which is higher above the desert floor than the North Window. This positioning invites us to climb up to the base of the opening to see what view awaits. Again, the scenery stretches across the desert mesas, and the large area beneath the arch is a popular photo stop.

Continuing on the clockwise loop, you'll descend westward in the direction of Turret Arch. Turret Arch is set within a staunch fin that is more than 100 feet wide. The opening to the arch is 64 feet high and 39 feet wide, making it the smallest of the three arches. By scrambling up inside the arch, you can capture a photo of the Windows framed by Turret Arch.

Completing the loop, you'll return to the parking area in a couple of minutes. But for an alternate, slightly longer return, consider the primitive loop trail, which starts at the South Window viewpoint and makes a counterclockwise loop behind the Windows, offering a rare view of Turret Arch framed by the North Window.

TO THE TRAILHEAD

GPS Coordinates: N38º 41.227' W109º 33.197'

From the Arches National Park entrance station, continue on Arches Scenic Drive (the main park road) for 8.9 miles to the road signed for the Windows section. Turn right and follow The Windows Road for 2.6 miles to the loop parking area at the end of the road.

HOW DO THE ARCHES FORM?

Arches form in a variety of ways. The ones in Arches National Park got their start some 300 million years ago, when a thick salt bed was deposited over the area. Residue from marine sediments was deposited on top of this salt bed, and

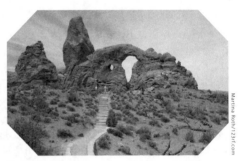

Turret Arch

eventually it compressed and hardened to rock. The weight of the rock put strain on the salt bed, causing it to become unstable and reposition itself, which in turn caused the overlaying rock to settle, forming domes and cavities. Over time, wind and water have created openings in the rock, which are now delicate and beautiful arches.

4 Double Arch

Trailhead Location: In the Windows section, on the north side of the Double Arch parking area

Trail Use: Walking, hiking

Distance & Configuration: 0.6-mile out-and-back

Elevation Range: 5,132' at trailhead to 5,210' within the arch

Facilities: Vault toilet near trailhead

Highlights: An easy, short walk to the second-largest arch in the park, which is also one of the most intriguing

DESCRIPTION

Double Arch is a spectacular sight and one of the most popular arches in the park. Because of its fame, if you want to have it to yourself, consider making this an early-morning or late-afternoon stop. Even if this is your first visit to Arches, you may remember seeing this arch before in the

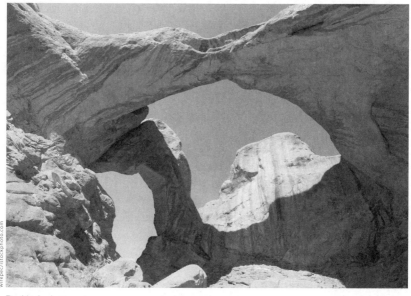

Double Arch

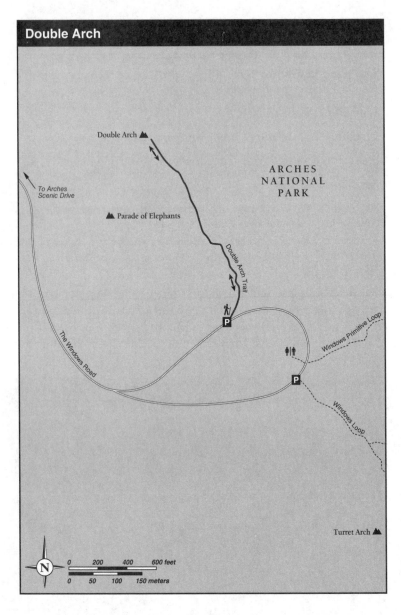

Double Arch

Double Arch ▲▲

ARCHES
NATIONAL
PARK

To Arches
Scenic Drive

▲▲ Parade of Elephants

Double Arch Trail

The Windows Road

Windows Primitive Loop

Windows Loop

Turret Arch ▲▲

0   200   400   600 feet

0   50   100   150 meters

N

opening scene of *Indiana Jones and the Last Crusade*. But don't bother looking for the treasure-laden cave nearby—that was pure Hollywood.

The eastern arch (the one closest to the trailhead) is 104 feet high and
148 feet wide, as measured with high-tech laser equipment in 2009, while

the smaller, more circular western arch is 60 feet by 60 feet. No guardrails or fences keep you from exploring underneath and around the arches, so enjoy them to your heart's content.

ROUTE

From the well-marked trailhead, the route descends slightly and heads directly toward the arch, with only a small amount of undulation and weaving. You must contend with some sand, but the trail is an easy jaunt suitable for all hikers. Along this flat you'll see junipers and oaks, with wildflowers in the spring, including Utah's state flower, the sego lily, with its large, three-petaled white flower. Indigenous peoples roasted sego lily bulbs or cooked them in stews. Later, Mormon pioneers ate the bulbs during their first years in Utah, especially in times of drought or crop failure.

To the left side of the trail you'll see a formation called the Parade of Elephants. Most people will comment on the elephant-shaped rocks before even knowing the name—it's that obvious.

When you arrive at Double Arch and enter into the chamber of the two arches, you might feel as though you're inside one of those mind-bending, impossible M. C. Escher etchings. Look up and around—are there two arches or three? If you count the top opening as an arch, you could call this Triple Arch, but actually, the top opening is not an arch, though it is instrumental in the forming of Double Arch.

Double Arch is defined as a pothole arch because it was formed by water erosion from above, so the arch overhead is where the water settled that then seeped down and began the formation of the arch, first by creating large alcoves and then by breaking through to complete the full arch. Most other arches form from the side.

Once you've wrapped your mind around this geologic puzzle, you can make your way back to the parking lot the way you came.

TO THE TRAILHEAD

GPS Coordinates: N38º 41.299' W109º 32.301'
From the Arches National Park entrance station, continue on Arches Scenic Drive (the main park road) for 8.9 miles to the road signed for the Windows section. Turn right and follow The Windows Road for 2.6 miles to the loop parking area at the end of the road. The Double Arch Trailhead is on the north side of the parking area.

WHERE ARE THE LEAVES ON
THE MORMON TEA SHRUB?

While inspecting the Mormon tea shrub, also known as ephedra, you may see a lot of naked, jointed, green branches. Look closely at the joints; you'll find tiny scalelike leaves. If you're observing the plant between February and April, you may even find small flowers blooming. Mormon tea, a mild stimulant and diuretic, was prized for its medicinal properties by both ancient inhabitants and early settlers. (*Note:* This species of ephedra is different from the kind that was 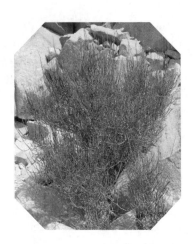 banned by the Food and Drug Administration as an ingredient in over-the-counter health supplements.)

5 Delicate Arch

Trailhead Location: Wolfe Ranch parking area in the heart of the park

Trail Use: Walking, hiking

Distance & Configuration: 3.0-mile out-and-back

Elevation Range: 4,307' at the Delicate Arch parking area to 4,841' at Delicate Arch

Facilities: Pit toilets at trailhead; no water

Highlights: The most iconic natural arch in the world

DESCRIPTION

If you have just one day in Arches National Park and time to hike just one trail, then a pilgrimage to Delicate Arch, the landmark symbol for Utah and the desert Southwest, is the must-do hike in the park. You'll cross a desert wash, ascend an impressive span of slickrock, and enjoy commanding views along the way. But none of that can prepare you for the surprise that awaits you at the end of the trail as this freestanding geologic masterpiece suddenly appears in majestic splendor.

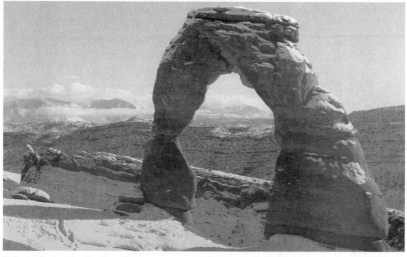

Delicate Arch with a dusting of snow

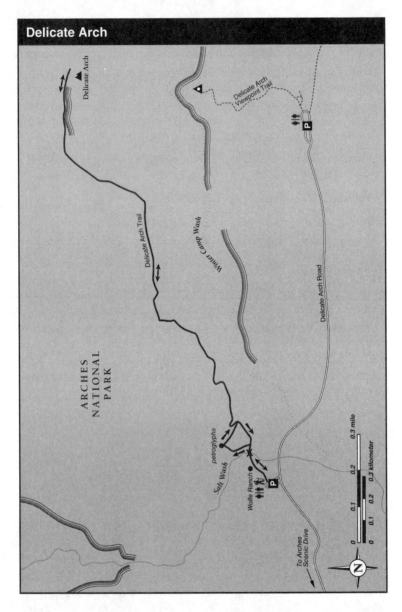

Delicate Arch

Delicate Arch

Delicate Arch Viewpoint Trail

Delicate Arch Trail

Winter Camp Wash

Delicate Arch Road

ARCHES NATIONAL PARK

petroglyphs

Salt Wash

Wolfe Ranch

To Arches Scenic Drive

0.3 mile

0.3 kilometer

But don't go unprepared—the shadeless route can be especially drain-ing in the summer sun. Take at least a half-gallon of water per person, and allow ample time to enjoy the arch and return to the trailhead parking area before nightfall. Because this hike is especially popular in the late afternoon, you'll want to check and see when the sun sets, so you can make it back safely. And because there's no water at the trailhead, you'd be wise to fill a few jugs at the visitor center on your way into the park.

ROUTE

As you depart the trailhead parking area on a wide, groomed path heading south, the first attraction is Wolfe Ranch, on your left. The weathered timbers of the old cabin are still sturdy and stand as a tribute to the tenacity and a reminder of the hardship of those who scratched out an existence in this harsh desert climate. Wolfe Ranch, settled in 1888 and abandoned in 1910, was the only homestead ever established in what is now Arches National Park. As you cross a sturdy metal bridge over Salt Wash, which at this point is a perennial alkaline trickle near the cabin, you'll wonder how or why anyone would have chosen a life in this remote outpost.

Crossing a stretch of greasewood desert, you'll see a short spur trail on the left heading over to American Indian petroglyphs. These are relatively modern, about 200 years old, compared to the much older Fremont and ancestral Puebloan rock art in other national parks in Utah. The presence of riders on horseback in these petroglyphs easily identifies them as Ute; it wasn't until contact with Spanish explorers in the late 18th century that Utah tribes acquired horses.

At 0.2 mile from the trailhead, your first major elevation gain begins with two switchbacks. The path brings you to the crest of a mound before dropping into a swale. In front of you is a band of Navajo Sandstone cliffs, as well as some arches in the making.

At the top of the steps you begin the longest ascending stretch of the hike across a steeply graded barren slickrock face. It's a straightforward ascent, and you'll certainly have company on the trail, so the lack of cairns shouldn't be a concern.

Reaching the top of the slickrock incline at 1.1 miles from the trailhead, the trail bends to the left and enters a maze of fins, where the trail is marked by cairns and caped by junipers.

Emerging from the fin maze, the trail opens up a bit, but you must still follow the cairns. Note the sweeping lines of the bowl to your left, where the walls are pockmarked by erosion. The trail continues on and veers to the right.

Your final approach to Delicate Arch takes you onto a catwalk ledge with some steep drop-offs on the left. It's safe and comfortable hiking on a bed of solid sandstone, but be sure to keep young children close at hand.

Instantly, at the end of the ledge trail and exactly 1.5 miles from the trailhead, the wall to your right drops and Delicate Arch comes into full view. It's easy to spend an hour or more at the arch, which invites both contemplation and photographs. Although most people sit across the bowl from the arch and enjoy it at a distance, you're certainly free to walk over to and directly under the arch and take photos from any angle you wish.

As you return the way you came, you can take the spur to the right and visit the petroglyphs. This short spur adds just a few minutes and less than 0.1 mile to your return.

TO THE TRAILHEAD
GPS Coordinates: N38° 44.140' W109° 35.230'
From the Arches National Park entrance station, drive 11.7 miles on Arches Scenic Drive to Wolfe Ranch–Delicate Arch Viewpoint Road. Turn right and drive 1.2 miles to the parking area on the left.

WOLFE RANCH

In 1888 John Wesley Wolfe, still nursing a leg injury from the Civil War, left Ohio in search of a drier climate that might provide some relief from his chronic pain. The desert of southeastern Utah seemed like a good choice. With his oldest son, Fred, he picked 100-plus acres along Salt Wash, where he would have a perennial, though limited, supply of water and grassland for a few cattle. They built a one-room cabin and corral, along with a small dam on Salt Wash. They lived alone at Wolfe Ranch for more than a decade. In 1906 John's daughter Flora, along with her husband and children, moved to the ranch. Shocked at the primitive living conditions, Flora and her family constructed the cabin with a wood floor that

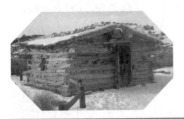

you see today—an upgrade from the previous dirt floor. The family moved to Moab in 1908, selling the ranch in 1910. John returned to Ohio and died in 1913 at the age of 84.

6 Delicate Arch Viewpoint

Trailhead Location: Delicate Arch Viewpoint parking area

Trail Use: Walking, hiking, wheelchair-accessible for first 100 yards to Lower Viewpoint

Distance & Configuration: 1.4-mile out-and-back

Elevation Range: 4,356' at trailhead to 4,510' at Upper Delicate Arch Viewpoint

Facilities: Pit toilets at trailhead; no water

Highlights: The easy way to see Delicate Arch from a distance

DESCRIPTION

Imagine that you've had a full day at Arches; it's late in the afternoon, everyone is tired and hungry, and there's no water in the car. You've seen the Windows, Double Arch, and Devils Garden. You have just 20 minutes remaining in the park, and not enough time, energy, or water to hike the Delicate Arch Trail. You know you could never forgive yourself if you left without seeing Delicate Arch, so what do you do?

If you can't hike the 3.0-mile Delicate Arch Trail, a short walk to Delicate Arch Viewpoint is a good plan B. Nothing matches the drama and majesty of seeing Delicate Arch face-to-face. But from this trail you'll see Delicate Arch just a quarter mile in the distance—close enough that you can return home and say, "I saw Delicate Arch." And no doubt, this tantalizing glimpse will whet your appetite for a return visit.

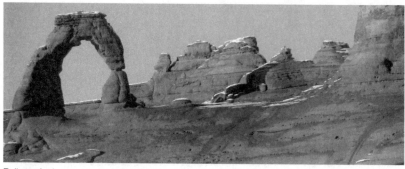

Delicate Arch

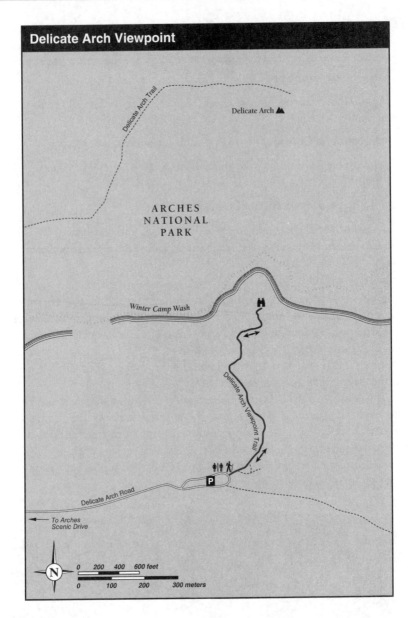

Delicate Arch Viewpoint

Delicate Arch Trail

Delicate Arch ▲▲

ARCHES
NATIONAL
PARK

Winter Camp Wash

Delicate Arch Viewpoint Trail

Delicate Arch Road

To Arches
Scenic Drive

N

| 0 | 200 | 400 | 600 feet |
| 0 | 100 | 200 | 300 meters |

ROUTE

From the east side of the large parking area, the trail heads east on a nicely graded, wide, compacted trail with a light gravel surface. This initial section of the trail is wheelchair- and stroller-accessible, and leads to an interpretive sign and a distant view of Delicate Arch.

From this junction, continue east on what was once a road leading to a viewpoint but now crosses slickrock patches of junipers on a route with cairns as your guide. The path continues, with intermittent views of the arch, toward a ridge, with Winter Camp Wash separating you from Delicate Arch. At 0.7 mile from the trailhead, you reach the Upper Viewpoint and a 200-foot drop-off into the wash below—an impressive view in its own right. Because most of the photos of Delicate Arch are from the Delicate Arch Trail and picture the other side of the arch, what you're seeing is really a different perspective; still, you get the effect of the arch's beauty and solitary position.

Backtrack the way you came, an easy downhill jaunt.

TO THE TRAILHEAD

GPS Coordinates: N38° 44.047' W109° 30.070'

From the Arches National Park entrance station, drive 11.7 miles on Arches Scenic Drive to Wolfe Ranch–Delicate Arch Viewpoint Road. Turn right and drive 1.2 miles to the spur road leading to Wolfe Ranch. Continue straight ahead for another 1.0 mile to the end of the road and the Delicate Arch Viewpoint parking area.

RATTLESNAKES

Although these venomous snakes are widely feared when spotted on the trail, rattlesnakes are vital to the desert ecosystem. They help control the rodent population and are food for other animals as well. Eight rattlesnake subspecies live in Utah. The most common is the Great Basin rattlesnake, found across the state. You might also come across the midget faded rattlesnake, a subspecies native to Arches. This snake grows to less than 2 feet long, is mainly active in the evenings, and lives in rock crevasses and burrows. If it sees you, this shy species will usually try to get out of your way. It does have a venomous bite, so if you see one of these local reptilian residents, it's best to respect and enjoy this beautiful desert creature from a safe distance. Also remember that rattlesnakes are protected by Utah law and within the national park; it is illegal to harass or kill a rattlesnake.

7 Fiery Furnace

Trailhead Location: Fiery Furnace Viewpoint parking area

Trail Use: Walking, hiking

Distance & Configuration: Approximate 2.0-mile hike

Elevation Range: 4,766' at trailhead with typical elevation gain/loss of 200'–300'

Facilities: Vault toilet at trailhead

Highlights: A labyrinth of fins and slots, secret passageways, and impossible dead-ends—an Arches treasure

DESCRIPTION

The name Fiery Furnace comes not from the scorching summer sun—actually, you'll find plenty of shade here—but from the fiery red hues of the rock and the flamelike contour of the sandstone fins. The Fiery Furnace is compact—less than a mile long and never more than 0.5 mile wide. But in that maze of tightly formed fins, it's easy to get lost, or at least briefly disoriented. That's why hikers must join a guided hike or obtain a special permit to enter Fiery Furnace. The rule is as much for the protection of the native plants and soils as it is for the safety of inexperienced hikers. If you've never hiked in Fiery Furnace previously, it is strongly recommended that you join a ranger-led hike.

During the busy season, rangers lead 3-hour, moderately strenuous hikes through the Fiery Furnace. Tickets for this guided hike must be obtained in advance for a fee. But remember that the rangers are guides, not Seeing Eye dogs, so you'll still need to take a measure of personal responsibility and preparation. Wear good hiking shoes with gripping soles; no sandals or high-heeled shoes are allowed. Each hiker must bring at least 1 quart of water carried in a small pack with your other gear, so your hands are free to navigate some often-challenging terrain.

On the guided hike you need to traverse narrow ledges with steep drop-offs, do some basic climbing maneuvers on irregular and broken sandstone, and be able to jump across gaps and fissures between the fins. Once you enter the Fiery Furnace, each member of the guided group must commit to complete the hike. Because of these demands, children younger than age 5

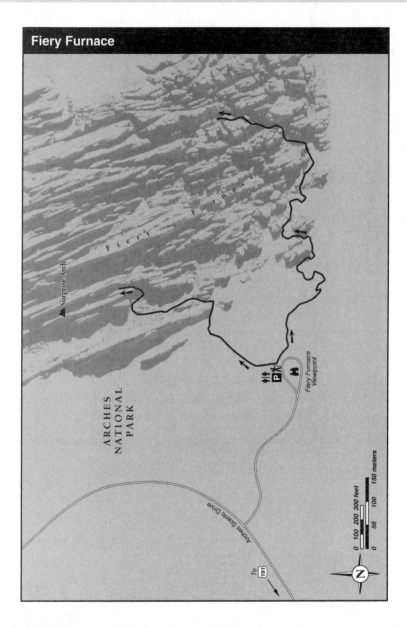

are not permitted, and children younger than 12 must be accompanied by an adult. Tickets for joining the guided hike may be purchased in advance on the park's website, **nps.gov/arch**.

ROUTE

Fiery Furnace is a uniquely Arches experience, a hike with no trail, no route, no cairns, no destination, no map, and no signs—in short, there's nothing like it anywhere else in the park.

If you've previously hiked Fiery Furnace with a guided group and completed a training session at the visitor center, you may be issued a special-use permit to enter Fiery Furnace as an independent hiker, but you are strongly encouraged to go with a ranger-guided group whenever possible.

If you're on your own, you can make your descent into the Fiery Furnace from either the northeast or southeast side of the parking area. Along any of the three well-beaten trails you'll arrive at the fringe of the Fiery Furnace within 200 yards. Once you've entered, the parking area and trailhead are out of view, so you'll need to rely on a keen sense of direction to find your way back.

If you do get disoriented or lost, the best advice is to head in a westerly direction, which will ensure that you cross the Arches Scenic Drive at some point rather than wandering off into the desert. But just walking west is more easily said than done, because all the fins in the Fiery Furnace run northwest–southeast and create a significant barrier to crosswise travel.

TO THE TRAILHEAD

GPS Coordinates: N38º 44.594' W109º 33.948'

From the Arches Visitor Center, drive 14.5 miles along Arches Scenic Drive to the Fiery Furnace Viewpoint parking area on the right.

HOW DO FINS FORM?

The fins in Arches National Park formed from forces above and below the surface. A thick layer of subsurface salt buckled and liquefied, causing the overlaying rocks to shift. Above the surface, wind and water eroded and carved the rock. Water that seeped into cracks froze, expanded, and broke off chunks. The cracks continued to expand, creating fins, the product of a harsh and active desert environment.

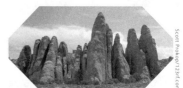

The majestic fins of Fiery Furnace

8 Sand Dune Arch and Broken Arch

Trailhead Location: Sand Dune Arch parking area

Trail Use: Walking, hiking

Distance & Configuration: 1.8-mile balloon with a short spur to Sand Dune Arch

Elevation Range: 5,192' at Sand Dune Arch Trailhead to 5,300' at Broken Arch

Facilities: Restrooms and water near the trail at Devils Garden Campground near Broken Arch

Highlights: Two very different arches accessed by a level path starting from either the parking area or the campground

DESCRIPTION

This hike starts at the Sand Dune Arch parking area, which is where most visitors arriving by car would logically start. But if you're staying inside the park at the Devils Garden Campground—a phenomenal campground, by the way—then leave the car behind and start your hike at the trailhead at campsite 40, at the south end of the campground.

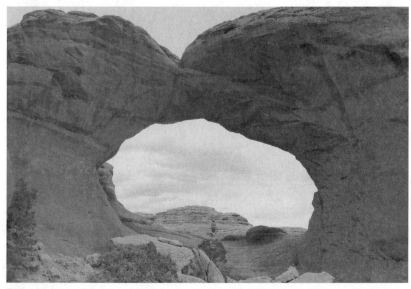

Broken Arch

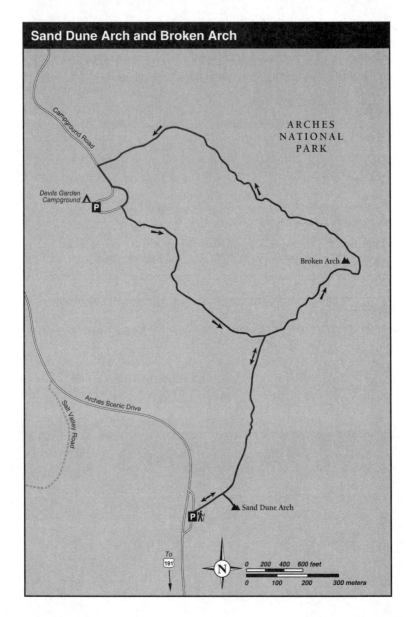

The hike features two arches with completely different personalities. One is a very private arch, small, reclusive, shy, and hidden from view—that's Sand Dune Arch. The other, Broken Arch, is big and bold, fully open to public view, and quite flashy. These personality differences can perhaps best be explained by their very different childhoods. Sand Dune was protected from outside influences and has led a sheltered life. Broken Arch came from a broken home. It has taken a real beating and has always had to fend for itself against the ravages of wind and rain. By hiking to both, you can discover which personality you're most compatible with, the introvert arch or the extrovert arch.

Along the way and between the two arches, you'll walk through desert brush dominated by sage, blackbrush, and some hardy grasses. It's a harsh environment, to be sure, with not a lick of shade between the two arches, so you might want to save this for cooler weather. It's also a great wake-up walk before breakfast for those staying at the campground.

ROUTE

Starting from the Sand Dune Arch parking area, the trail cuts through a sandy desert sparsely decorated with sagebrush, Mormon tea, and Indian ricegrass. At 100 yards you come to a junction with Broken Arch on the left, visible in the distance, and Sand Dune Arch, hidden from view but set within the mound of fins just 100 yards to your right. As you take the trail to the right toward Sand Dune Arch, the sand seems to deepen with every step you take. Entering what feels like a hallway—a crack set between two large walls of sandstone—you'll find that the base is one giant sandbox with some exposed slickrock made slippery by the fine layer of sand on top. Within seconds, you meet Sand Dune Arch face-to-face on your right. It's 30 feet wide and 8 feet high in a shaded setting.

Returning to the main trail, turn right and continue northeast toward Broken Arch. Walking on a sandy trail across a grassy brushland, you'll arrive at Broken Arch in less than 0.5 mile. Despite its name, the arch isn't really broken, but a deep cleft in the top of the arch makes it appear to be cut in two, or broken, at the top. But don't worry; it has plenty of life left.

While it's easy to leave shy Sand Dune Arch without ever taking its picture, bold Broken Arch demands to be photographed. Don't resist. In fact, using the arch as a frame, you'll have views of the Uncompahgre Plateau and the La Sal Mountains to the southeast. Broken Arch is 50 feet high and 60 feet wide—one of the largest arches in the park. Be sure to walk through the arch; you'll find that it's just as photogenic from its back or eastern side. From the backside of the arch, you have two options for returning to the parking area: You can hook to the left to connect with the trail leading to Devils Garden Campground and back to the parking area, or you can return the way you came, across the desert to the Sand Dune Arch parking area.

TO THE TRAILHEAD

GPS Coordinates: N38º 35.887' W109º 35.000'

The Sand Dune Arch parking area is 17.5 miles from the Arches Visitor Center on Arches Scenic Drive.

BIGHORN SHEEP

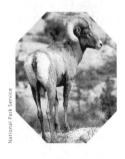

National Park Service

Bighorn sheep are native to North America. They are distinguished by their large, curved horns, which weigh up to 30 pounds and can be approximately one-tenth of their total body weight. The sheep's diet mainly consists of native grasses, sedges, and forbs. During the winter months, bighorn sheep get all their water from the plants they eat. In the summer, they need a drink of water only every three to four days. You will commonly find them in herds of 8–10.

It's common to see bighorn sheep butting heads and horns in a ritual that has more to do with establishing the dominant male within the group than just playfully showing off. In fact bighorn sheep can often butt heads at speeds up to 20 miles per hour. They have a two-layered cranium, with a cushy foamlike tissue between, that enables the sheep to survive that kind of concussion.

9 Devils Garden

Trailhead Location: Devils Garden Trailhead, at the end of Arches Scenic Drive

Trail Use: Walking, hiking

Distance & Configuration: 1.6-mile out-and-back to Landscape Arch; 4.0-mile out-and-back to Double O Arch; 5.4-mile out-and-back to Dark Angel; 7.2-mile balloon visiting all the arches and returning on the primitive trail

Elevation Range: 5,240' at trailhead with minor descent to Pine Tree Arch at 5,215' and gentle ascent to Landscape Arch at 5,256'

Facilities: Restrooms and water at trailhead

Highlights: Lots of arches in a compact area, including Landscape Arch, the longest in the world

DESCRIPTION

With so many prominent arches along the route, it's no surprise that Devils Garden is one of the most heavily used trail networks in the park. But all this attention is very much deserved, so don't let the crowds keep you away. You'll be rewarded with not only nine headliner arches but also a trail that courses its way between immense fins. The trail then ascends those fins to offer some of the best panoramic views in the park.

Devils Garden is really a collection of arches, like a giant museum with various galleries. You can peruse them all or pick and choose the ones that interest you most. The showstopper here—the *Mona Lisa* of Devils Garden—is Landscape Arch, one of the longest stone spans in the world, stretching 309 feet from wall to wall. That it's still standing after a 60-foot slab of rock fell from the underside of the arch's thinnest section in 1991 is miraculous. Today, Landscape Arch is only 11 feet thick at its center.

A popular park myth states that Landscape and Delicate Arches had their names mistakenly swapped by an errant cartographer. As with many myths, it does seem like a reasonable assumption, because the ribbon of stone in Landscape Arch really is more delicate than the solid flank of stone rising above the landscape in Delicate Arch.

For avid hikers, some of the most rewarding hiking in the park occurs after passing Landscape Arch on the way to Double O Arch. Here the

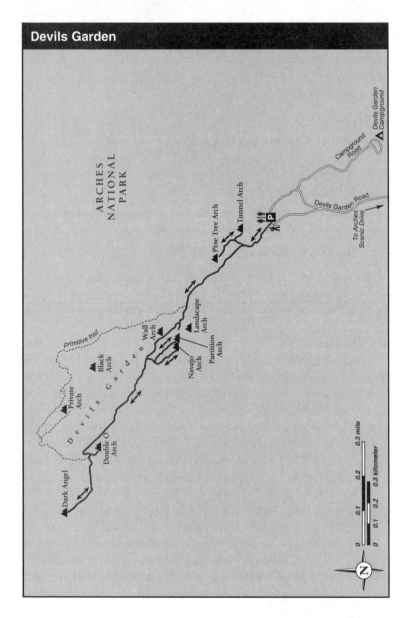

Devils Garden

ARCHES NATIONAL PARK

Devils Garden Campground

Campground Road

Devils Garden Road

To Arches Scenic Drive

Pine Tree Arch

Tunnel Arch

P

Landscape Arch

Wall Arch

Partition Arch

Navajo Arch

Black Arch

primitive trail

Private Arch

Devils Garden

Double O Arch

Dark Angel

0.3 mile

0.3 kilometer

0.1   0.2

0   0.1   0.2

0

N

route demands a little more attention, including following cairns and
watching for more-subtle trail markings such as footprints in the sand or
indented footholds on steep slickrock faces. You'll also face steep slickrock
surfaces leading to the top of a fin, which may require the use of both hands

and feet. Once on top of the fin, you'll have not only great views but also treacherous drop-offs on both sides.

If you make it as far as Double O Arch and still have a thirst for more adventure, consider the optional return along the primitive trail, forming a clockwise loop back to the main trail. Hiking the entire Devils Garden Trail, including the primitive trail, takes 3 hours or more. The primitive trail has almost no signage, and it's easy to get lost on its winding and varied course. Even if you have a good native sense of direction, you'll need to pay close attention, and don't even consider hiking the primitive trail when snow or ice cover the route.

ROUTE

Departing the trailhead on the wide, evenly graded, and well-compacted path, you quickly enter a joint between two immense fins, which often becomes a wind tunnel, so hold on to your hat. Emerging from the chasm onto a sandy flat dotted with sagebrush and Mormon tea, you'll soon come to a junction at 0.3 mile, with a signed spur on the right leading to Pine Tree Arch (just 0.2 mile down the spur) and Tunnel Arch, about 100 yards to the right on the same spur. Pine Tree Arch spans an area 46 feet wide by 48 feet high and is one of the few arches in the park set at ground level.

Continuing another 0.5 mile on the main trail past the junction, you come to a rise, with your first glimpse of Landscape Arch in the distance to the northwest. Continue on the main trail to the short spur on the left leading to Landscape Arch, and once at the end of the spur, be sure to stay within the confines of the fence.

Beyond Landscape Arch, the trail becomes more rugged and less defined in places, climbing between and over a fin onto piñon–juniper benchland. Signs point to Partition Arch and Navajo Arch on a spur to the left. Once on the spur, each arch is accessed by its own sub-spur to the left. First comes Partition Arch, set on a wall with an opening about 26 feet wide and 28 feet high. Returning to the main spur and continuing to the left, you'll arrive at Navajo Arch in 0.2 mile. Navajo Arch is a gracefully formed semicircle about 41 feet wide and 13 feet high.

Returning to the main trail, you'll soon mount a fin, which often requires a boost from a companion hiker or stepping onto a log ramp. Once on top of the fin, you'll have some of the best long-range views in the park across Salt Valley and beyond.

Soon your route atop the fin descends and offers a jumping-off point to the left. Following footsteps through the sand amid a mazelike cluster of small fins shaded by piñons and junipers, you'll encounter Double O Arch almost by surprise. Double O is a tough arch to photograph because it's one arch on top of the other at a close range, but it's a great place to stop for lunch in one of the many shaded nooks nearby.

From the cozy confines of Double O Arch, you have several options. You can return to the parking area the way you came; you can proceed to Dark Angel, which adds another mile to the trip; or you can also follow the signs to the primitive trail. The signs warn of difficult hiking, and though the primitive trail is really no more physically demanding than what you've already encountered on your way from Landscape Arch, it does require a higher level of route-finding skill. But with ample water, some extra time, and a little patience, you'll certainly enjoy the primitive trail return.

TO THE TRAILHEAD
GPS Coordinates: N38° 46.978' W109° 35.707'
From the Arches Visitor Center drive 17.5 miles on Arches Scenic Drive to the Devils Garden parking area. The trailhead is on the north side of the parking-area loop.

WHAT QUALIFIES AS AN ARCH?

In Arches National Park there are more than 2,500 arches of various sizes and shapes. But what does it take to be officially classified an arch? Can any hole in a rock be given that distinguished designation?

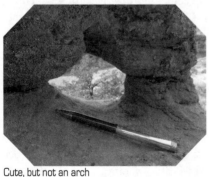
Cute, but not an arch

Absolutely not. But there is no general consensus among geologists about how big an arch must be to qualify as a named and cataloged arch within Arches National Park. Early in the park's history, one official suggested that an arch must have a span of at least 10 feet in any direction. Today, park publications state that a hole in the rock must have an opening of at least 3 feet.

10 Tower Arch

Trailhead Location: Accessed by a dirt road leading through Salt Valley to the Klondike Bluffs area of the park

Trail Use: Walking, hiking

Distance & Configuration: 3.4-mile out-and-back

Elevation Range: 5,082' at trailhead to 5,512' at Tower Arch

Facilities: Vault toilet at trailhead

Highlights: A hike through the varied terrain of the Klondike Bluffs to a remote and beautifully cut arch

DESCRIPTION

This moderately strenuous hike leads to Tower Arch, a spectacular formation nestled among the fractured rock of the Klondike Bluffs. Today, the Klondike Bluffs section of Arches National Park is a remote region rarely explored by most park visitors. But for most of the past century, Klondike Bluffs was the first exposure many visitors had to Arches because the only vehicle access to the park before the 1960s was through the Salt Valley.

In 1922 Hungarian-born prospector Alex Ringhoffer first invited railroad executives to Klondike Bluffs, at the time called Devils Garden, in an attempt to interest them in the area's tourism potential. Soon thereafter a steady stream of other journalists, reporters, and National Park Service officials began to take interest in the unusual spires, arches, and rock formations in the area, leading President Herbert Hoover to sign the declaration creating Arches National Monument in 1929. As you visit Tower Arch, look for the inscription under the arch referencing Ringhoffer, but please don't touch.

As the region was being explored and mapped, there was some confusion regarding the names in the area, and the name Devils Garden was mistakenly assigned to the area east of Salt Valley, where that name remains in use today. The name for the original Devils Garden was then changed to Klondike Bluffs.

ROUTE

The trail to Tower Arch offers hikers a good challenge and a worthy reward for the effort. The first challenge comes just seconds from the trailhead, as

Tower Arch

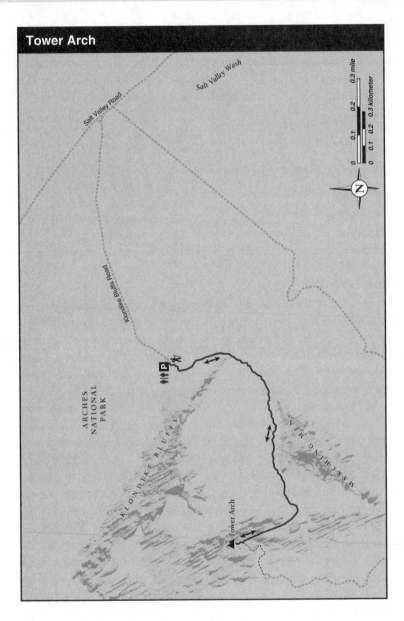

you make an ascent through steep and rock-strewn slabs of slickrock to cross over and through Klondike Bluffs. The trail isn't always easy to follow, as it takes you by surprise with a number of hairpin turns, but at 0.2 mile you arrive at the crest of the bluff with captivating views to the east and west.

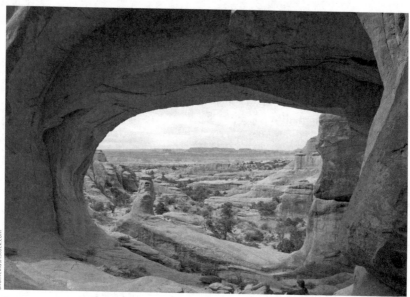

Tower Arch

The trail then makes an easy descent into a small swale at about 0.4 mile from the trailhead and finally arrives at the main wash at 0.9 mile. *Important:* Trail signage is sparse, and you'll see footprints heading down the wash to the left, but do not follow them. Instead, cross the wash with a slight jog to the right in the direction of the cairn.

After crossing the wash, the trail rises steeply through sand in the direction of the north fins of the Klondike Bluffs. This sand is so fine that you'll want to take off your shoes and run your toes through it, but it will work its way into your shoes and socks without your even removing them.

Now atop the sandy slope, you'll pass through a level stretch of the Dewey Bridge formation, with Entrada Sandstone fins towering above. Then, at 0.4 mile from the wash, you arrive at the base of magnificent Tower Arch. You'll want to bask in its shade and take photos of companions framed by it.

The inscription in stone under the arch, DISCOV'D BY M. AND MRS. ALEX RINGHOEFFER AND SONS IN 1922–3, raises questions such as, "Was this written by Alex Ringhoffer?" and "If so, why the uncertain date?" These and other questions will likely remain unanswered for as long as this sturdy arch remains standing.

After enjoying the splendor of this remote arch, you can return the way you came; the descent down the sandy hill should be much more enjoyable than your ascent.

TO THE TRAILHEAD

GPS Coordinates: N38° 47.549' W109° 40.518'

From the Arches Visitor Center, travel 16.7 miles along Arches Scenic Drive to the Salt Valley Road turn-off, on your left. Continue for 7.3 miles on the graded Salt Valley Road to a junction with a road going off to the left. Do not turn on this road, but continue for another 50 yards and turn left on the road signed to Klondike Bluffs at 1 mile. Continue west on this dirt road to the small circular parking area.

CHERT: NOT JUST ANOTHER PRETTY ROCK

Approximately 10,000 years ago, ancient inhabitants roamed the Colorado Plateau. They weren't sightseeing like the millions of visitors who come here today. Instead, they were in search of life-sustaining resources. One of those resources was chert, a microcrystalline quartz rock. A tough sedimentary rock that can be easily shaped into a sharp edge, chert was used to cut tools and craft weapon points, making it an important rock to ancient inhabitants. Archaeologists have found debris piles of this rock, remnants of ancient inhabitants knapping (chipping) the rock into valuable tools.

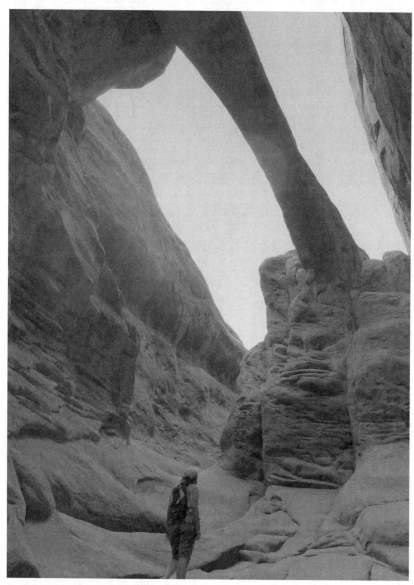

An arch in Fiery Furnace (see Hike 7, page 38)

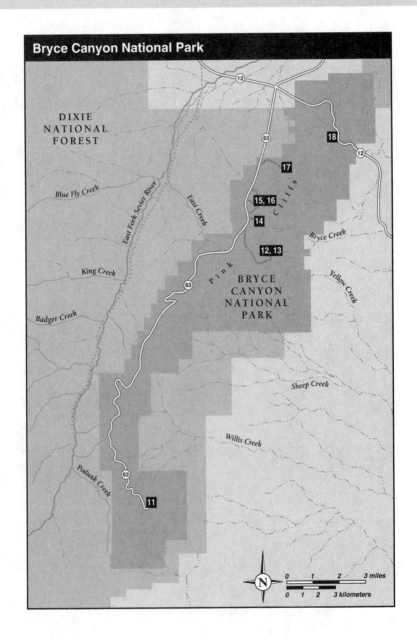

Bryce Canyon National Park

BRYCE CANYON NATIONAL PARK

Park Overview

Bryce Canyon is Utah's smallest national park—a glistening jewel cast in hues of yellow, pink, orange, and red. But its name is a misnomer because it isn't a canyon. Canyons are carved by rivers, while Bryce Canyon is actually a series of eroding cliffs on the eastern rim of the Paunsaugunt Plateau. The cliffs have formed brightly colored rock amphitheaters decorated with bizarrely shaped ridges, fins, and hoodoos. This otherworldly landscape, replete with windows, arches, and natural bridges, fuels the imagination and makes for irresistibly fun hiking.

Bryce is Utah's highest-elevation national park, and as in Utah's other national parks, you can read Earth's history in layers of stone. Geologically, Bryce can rightly be considered the uppermost rim of the Grand Canyon— a relatively young Cenozoic layer, softer and more quickly erodible than the formations found in other national parks in the Colorado Plateau. Because it's high and dry, you'll find an intriguing variety of alpine trees and shrubs in Bryce that are not found in the lower elevations of the Colorado Plateau.

Southern Paiutes and other American Indians lived in the area. But because of its higher elevation and less hospitable climate for growing crops, the immediate area that is now part of Bryce Canyon National Park was not as heavily populated as other parts of the Southwest were. Not until military men passed through the area in 1866 did it become known to the rest of America. In 1872 geologist G. K. Gilbert explored the area, and after first seeing the hoodoos, he wrote: "We caught a glimpse of a perfect wilderness of red pinnacles." Bryce Canyon became a national monument in 1923 and was designated as a national park in 1928.

JUST ONE DAY?

Bryce's small size and linear layout mean it can be easily visited in one day. Even if all you do is stop at the viewpoints on the rim, you can see a high percentage of the park. But the greatest hikes in Bryce lie below the rim and require you to lace up your boots and hit the trail.

Begin with a stop at the visitor center, and proceed by car or shuttle to Rainbow Point, on the park's southernmost rim, for a short walk on the Bristlecone Loop. Because all the viewpoints are on the east side of the road, stopping at them is most easily done on your northward return, thereby requiring no left turns. When you arrive at either Sunset or Sunrise Point, hike the 3-mile Queens Garden and Navajo Loop, which is not just the finest hike in the park but is also arguably the finest short hike in America.

◘ ◘ ◘

"A HELLUVA PLACE TO LOSE A COW"

That's how Ebenezer Bryce, a ship carpenter from Scotland, described the labyrinthine landscape of Bryce Canyon. After joining the Church of Jesus Christ of Latter-day Saints at the age of 17, he immigrated to Utah and helped settle the area in 1875. He is well known for his many contributions to the area. Such projects include building a road to the canyon to access timber more easily and helping construct a 7-mile-long irrigation canal. He was also known for building a Mormon chapel in nearby Pine Valley that is still used today. The people began calling the area "Bryce's Canyon," and the name stuck long after he moved away.

11 Bristlecone Loop

Trailhead Location: Rainbow Point parking area

Trail Use: Walking, hiking

Distance & Configuration: 1.0-mile loop

Elevation Range: 9,121' at trailhead to 9,145' along trail

Facilities: Restrooms and water at trailhead

Highlights: A loop through a dense fir forest entirely above the canyon rim

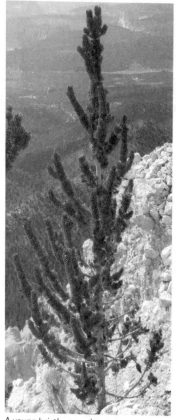

A young bristlecone pine

DESCRIPTION

Rainbow Point sits at the highest elevation within Bryce Canyon National Park. It's a harsh alpine environment—a windswept perch where only the strong survive. At the windiest point of the trail, where few other species endure, a bristlecone pine tree has lived for more than 1,600 years. This bristlecone's trunk has been dead for many years, but a surviving branch has become the main tree in a textbook example of how species adapt to even the most severe environments.

In this coldest extension of the park, most of the trees are white fir and Douglas-fir, in contrast to the ponderosa pines found on the lower plateaus. Here trees seek mutual support as they grow in dense stands and deep shade, so that their shadows prolong moisture-giving snowbanks and steal sunlight from competing species.

The Bristlecone Loop is a great starting hike in Bryce Canyon. Because the layout of Bryce Canyon consists of

Bristlecone Loop

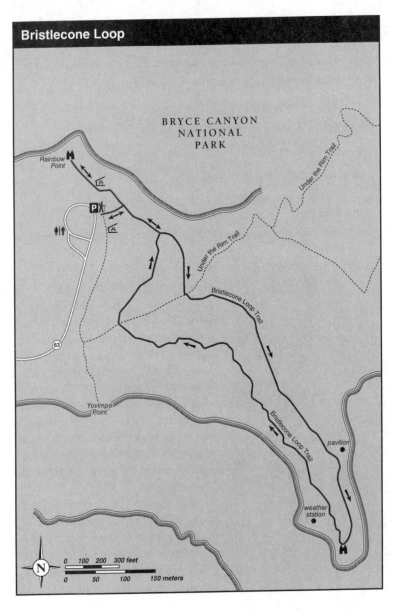

amphitheaters and viewpoints, all of which are on the east side of UT 63, one recommended strategy for visiting the park is to start your day by driving to Rainbow Point, at the southernmost and highest elevation in the park. Then pick off the viewpoints on your return to the park exit.

That way you traverse the entire park and never have to make a left turn—pretty smart.

The Bristlecone Loop is also unique within Bryce Canyon because it's the only hike in the park where trees, not geology, are the focus and theme of the hike. This short loop has more shade than most of the other trails in Bryce and, at this high elevation, also predictably cooler temperatures, so come prepared with an extra layer of warmth for this beautiful stroll through an alpine forest.

ROUTE

Start by heading west to the interpretive sign at the parking area, where the trail takes off to the south through a conifer forest cover. At 100 yards from the parking lot, you reach a signed junction marking the start of the Bristlecone Loop, which continues straight ahead and moves in a clockwise circuit. This junction also is the starting point for the Under the Rim Trail, an unforgettable 23-mile route set below the Pink Cliffs. It's a spectacular hike—one you'll definitely want to save for a return visit as a two-day backpacking trip.

The trail surface is wide, well graded, well defined, and edged the entire way. It would be wheelchair-accessible were it not for the occasional fallen tree crossing the trail, which requires a few big steps or straddles to get around. Along the trail, the sparse ground cover consists of manzanitas and stunted Oregon grapes.

At 0.5 mile you arrive at a viewpoint pavilion with interpretive signs. At this elevation, the highest in the park, the view almost seems aerial as you gaze down to the hoodoos and amphitheaters below—very different from the rim views in other parts of the park. Looking 30 miles to the east, you can see the Aquarius Plateau and the Kaiparowits Plateau. The Paunsaugunt Plateau where you now stand was once connected to the Aquarius Plateau. But about 16 million years ago, when the Rocky Mountains began their upward thrust, a north–south fault fractured the vast tableland into seven separate sections.

Moving on from the pavilion, the trail bends to the right to reach a second viewpoint on the southwest side of the promontory, with great scenery to the south and into Zion National Park, though none of Zion's iconic monuments are viewable from this distance or angle. This windy bluff is a favorite nesting area for peregrine falcons, which live in cliffside grottoes. These falcons revel in high winds and, in dramatic dives, reach speeds up to 200 miles per hour.

As the trail bends back to the north on its return, you pass a weather-observation station perched on a cliff to the left. Continuing as the trail gently winds through the forest, the loop trail technically ends at the junction with the Yovimpa Spur Trail at 0.8 mile, but your return to the parking area brings the total distance to 1.0 mile. Taking the Yovimpa Spur Trail to the left adds almost nothing to your time or distance and gives you an additional overlook, this time to the west. It's wheelchair-accessible and highly recommended. As you return to the parking area, be sure to make the short walk over to Rainbow Point. You've already had some great views on this trail, and this namesake viewpoint adds to the splendor.

TO THE TRAILHEAD

GPS Coordinates: N37º 28.459' W112º 14.417'
From the Bryce Canyon Visitor Center, drive 17.0 miles south on UT 63 to the trailhead sign on the south side of the Rainbow Point parking area.

BRISTLECONE PINE

As the longest-living tree in the world, the bristlecone pine has outlived many generations of human visitors. The bristlecone pines in Bryce Canyon are up to 1,800 years old. Some bristlecones in Utah are known to be close to 5,000 years old! The twisted look of the tree stems from the way it grows: As its roots become exposed, the parts of the tree that received nutrients from those roots will die as well. The bristlecone can also increase its chance of survival during droughts by shutting down metabolism to some of its branches. The remaining sections of the plant will continue to grow. Unlike other pine trees that shed their needles every few years, bristlecones have needles that can stay intact for more than 40 years.

---

12 Hat Shop

Trailhead Location: Bryce Point Trailhead

Trail Use: Walking, hiking

Distance & Configuration: 4.0-mile out-and-back

Elevation Range: 8,323' at Bryce Point Trailhead to 7,300' at the Hat Shop

Facilities: None

Highlights: Typical Bryce hoodoos with a twist: They're capped with dolomite limestone.

DESCRIPTION

The Hat Shop is rarely visited by the thousands of park visitors who tend to stay close to the comfort of the rim, so it's not uncommon to spend 2 hours on this trail and, once you descend about 100 feet below the rim, not see another soul. This hike puts you on the final leg of the Under the Rim Trail—one of the greatest long trails in the country, a 23-mile route from Rainbow Point to Bryce Point.

The route traverses a piñon forest below the Pink Cliffs before dropping through hoodoos and into a side canyon. Once at the Hat Shop, you'll see a textbook example of how hoodoos form: Softer layers of sandstone lie beneath angular capstones of dolomite limestone. In a process known as differential erosion, the sandstone erodes at a faster rate than the harder limestone, thereby creating the distinctive and improbably balanced "hats." Each hat acts as an umbrella for the hoodoo below and provides it with some protection from further and faster erosion.

ROUTE

From the north side of the parking area, descend the long, wide trail steps to the right, in the direction of the Hat Shop and Peekaboo Loop. At 0.1 mile you arrive at a signed trail junction, with the Peekaboo Loop connector descending to the left and the Hat Shop Trail (the final leg of the longer Under the Rim Trail) continuing straight ahead. Continue straight. The trail undulates across the rim, dotted with manzanitas and sparse but varied conifers, including Douglas-firs, piñon pines, and ponderosa pines.

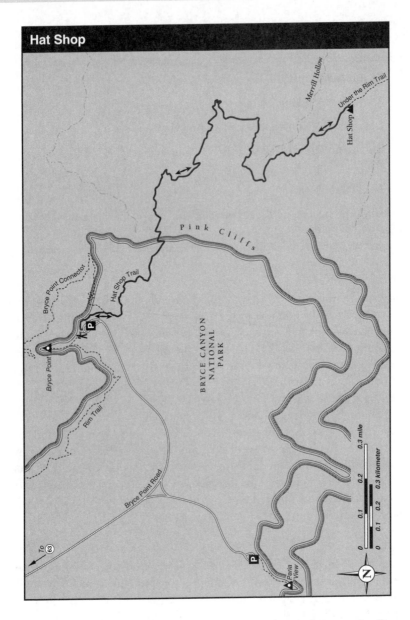

After this 0.5-mile stretch above the rim, the trail enters the Bryce Canyon Wilderness Area and begins its descent into the Pink Cliffs on steep switchbacks. Initially the trail is on the whitish layer of the Pink Cliffs, but it quickly enters the red section of the same formation. Shortly

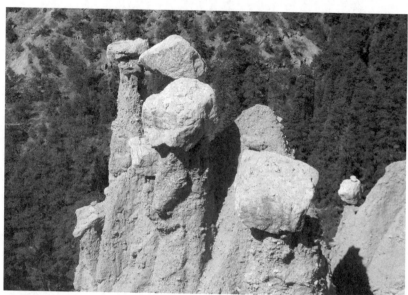

The Hat Shop

you're surrounded by Pink Cliff hoodoos and immersed in a very different ecosystem from the one you just experienced above the rim.

As you continue your descent, you arrive at a promontory about 1.5 miles from the trailhead. If you know what you're looking for, you'll get a glimpse of the Hat Shop in the distance to the south. But the more sweeping and compelling views are to the east, where the Aquarius Plateau on the left and Kaiparowits Plateau on the right stretch across the horizon, 40 miles or more in the distance.

Passing the promontory, the trail curves to the right and stays fairly level as it contours its way along a side canyon, initially moving to the northwest in the opposite direction of the Hat Shop before making a bend to the left for your final approach.

There is no sign marking the Hat Shop, so you'll need to pay attention to the hoodoos on the right side of the trail. At exactly 2.0 miles from the trailhead, the path makes a quick rise onto a promontory where, on your right, you'll see hoodoos topped with precariously perched dolomite capstones—the Hat Shop! You're in full exposed sunlight, and it may take some hunting to find a nearby tree large enough to offer sufficient shade for a picnic. From the Hat Shop, you can continue down the Under the Rim Trail and do some exploring in this piñon–juniper woodland before returning to the trailhead the way you came.

TO THE TRAILHEAD

GPS Coordinates: N37º 36.262' W112º 9.418'

From the Bryce Canyon National Park entrance and visitor center, drive south on UT 63 for 1.6 miles to Bryce Point Road, on your left. Turn left onto Bryce Point Road and continue for 1.3 miles to a fork with Paria View on the right and Bryce Point on the left. Bear left and continue for 0.6 mile to the large parking area and viewpoint.

STONE PEOPLE

The word *hoodoo* may seem like an unscientific, unofficial, or colloquial name for the distinctive spires found in Bryce and other parts of the Colorado Plateau, but it is indeed a technical term used by geologists. The difference between a hoodoo and a spire or pinnacle is that hoodoos have a variable thickness, sometimes described as a totem pole–shaped body, whereas a spire has a smoother, more tapered profile. This variable thickness occurs when a harder rock layer sits on top of a softer, more easily eroded layer.

According to ancient legend, hoodoos were believed to be people whom the god Coyote turned to stone for misbehaving. In the Paiute language, hoodoos were called legend people. If you use your imagination, you can almost see their faces.

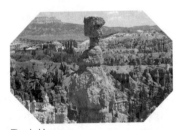
Thor's Hammer

13 Peekaboo Loop

Trailhead Location: Bryce Point Trailhead

Trail Use: Walking, hiking, horseback riding on one portion of the trail

Distance & Configuration: 4.9-mile balloon

Elevation Range: 8,300' at Bryce Point Trailhead to 7,450' at loop's farthest extension, near the signed junction

Facilities: Solar-composting toilet on Peekaboo Loop

Highlights: A superb loop hike below the rim through the southern half of the Bryce Amphitheater

DESCRIPTION

If Queens Garden is the best hike in Bryce Canyon National Park, then Peekaboo Loop must be a very close second. Think of Peekaboo Loop as a companion hike to Queens Garden and Navajo Loop—a longer, equally varied, and scenic hike to the south of Queens Garden. Peekaboo Loop plunges below the rim and winds through the hoodoos in the southern half of the Bryce Amphitheater in much the same way that the Queens Garden and Navajo Loop (page 72) explores the northern half of the amphitheater. Each hike is comprehensive in its approach and captures the most spectacular and noteworthy formations within its respective area.

The trail to Peekaboo Loop descends below the rim from Bryce Point via a short connecter. Once you're in the heart of the hoodoos, you'll be treated to some of Bryce Canyon's most iconic formations, including the Three Wise Men, the Cathedral, and the Organ. You'll also have eastward views to the Aquarius Plateau and the Kaiparowits Plateau.

On Peekaboo Loop you'll also pass the Wall of Windows, which may cause you to wonder, "What's the difference between a window and an arch?" In Utah's national parks, a hole in a fin can be designated as an arch or a window. Though there's no general agreement, some geologists suggest that an arch occurs at or near the base of a rock wall, like the doors of a house, whereas a window is found above ground level. Though the distinction is not always followed in the naming of the openings in Arches National Park, the Wall of Windows is a perfect example of a window rather than an arch, according to the above definition.

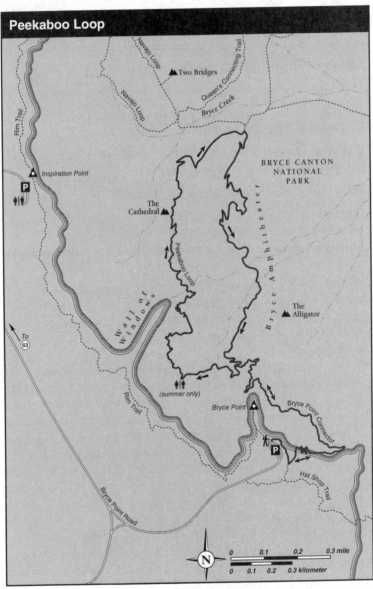

Because a portion of the loop is shared with horses, park officials rec-
ommend hiking the loop clockwise to avoid horses approaching hikers from
behind. The signage on the loop also supports that direction. Fortunately,
horse usage is light, so the trail is not too fouled, and the trail surface still
favors hikers.

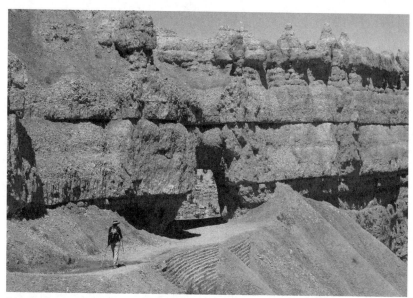
A hiker enjoying the delightful Peekaboo Loop

ROUTE

Your route below the rim starts with a quick descent along a steep but nicely groomed trail to a junction sign at 0.1 mile. Here you turn left onto the connector trail marked to Peekaboo Loop. The trail to the right leads to the Hat Shop, which you can save for another day.

The connector makes a quick descent into hoodoos along several sweeping switchbacks. Descending through scattered bristlecone and limber pines, you'll pass through a short man-made arch or small tunnel 0.5 mile from the trailhead. Here the views open up to the area in which you'll be hiking. Continuing your descent you'll arrive at the beginning of the loop within 1.0 mile from the trailhead.

Your first stop comes quickly as you arrive at the horse corral, with a picnic area and solar-composting toilet tucked in a shady spot to the left of the trail, making it a fine spot for a quick rest and snack.

Once you hit the loop, there's lots of undulation as you bob and weave your way under, around, and through the maze of hoodoos. At 0.3 mile from the start of the loop, you arrive at a viewpoint and sign directing your attention to the Wall of Windows, on the fin to the north.

At 1.1 miles on the loop, the trail completes its ascent and crests through a narrow passageway in the rock to move from the Bryce Amphitheater into the smaller amphitheater below Inspiration Point, with equally impressive views of the hoodoos—views, proximity, and perspective that drive-by tourists on the rim will never see. Consider yourself lucky.

At 1.9 miles on the loop, you'll come to the northerly extension of Peek-aboo Loop at one of the lowest elevations on the trail. You'll now begin your ascent on the return side—the east side of the loop—to complete the loop. After the initial steep ascent, the trail does some more winding, rising, and falling through especially scenic stretches of the Bryce Amphitheater to complete the loop in a total distance of just a little under 3.0 miles.

As you arrive at the same junction where you started the loop, turn left onto the connector trail for your ascent to the rim.

TO THE TRAILHEAD
GPS Coordinates: N37º 36.262' W112º 9.418'
From the Bryce Canyon National Park entrance and visitor center, drive south on UT 63 for 1.6 miles to Bryce Point Road, on your left. Turn left onto Bryce Point Road and continue for 1.3 miles to a fork with Paria View on the right and Bryce Point on the left. Bear left and continue for 0.6 mile to the large trailhead parking area and viewpoint.

HEY, WHO'S BAKING COOKIES?

While hiking through the canyons of southern Utah, you may get a whiff of freshly baked cookies, vanilla, or even cinnamon. Don't worry—you aren't losing your mind. That delicious smell is actually coming from a tree called the ponderosa pine. Widely distributed throughout the West, these trees can live up to 600 years and grow to an average height of 100–150 feet. When ponderosa pines are young, they have black bark. Once they reach the age of 100–120 years (a young age for a ponderosa), the black bark peels off, exposing the yellow, sweet-smelling bark that may remind you of a bakery. Go ahead; sniff the bark and enjoy.

14 Rim Trail

Trailhead Location: Sunset Point Trailhead

Trail Use: Walking, hiking, pets, wheelchair-accessible

Distance & Configuration: 1.0-mile out-and-back or 0.5-mile point-to-point

Elevation Range: 7,992' at Sunset Point Trailhead to 8,013' at Sunrise Point

Facilities: Restrooms, water, general store, and lodge near trailhead

Highlights: A connecting trail linking visitor services with the most popular viewpoints

DESCRIPTION

For many park visitors, a stroll along the Rim Trail, a night at the Bryce Canyon Lodge, and the view from the Sunrise and Sunset observation decks are the starting points for a Bryce Canyon vacation. And sadly, for some that's about the full extent of their visit. The area between Sunrise Point and Sunset Point is the traditional heart of the park, the location of the historic Bryce Canyon Lodge, the campgrounds, and the ranger office. It's a fine baseline, but use it as a gateway to the rest of the park's wonders.

The most popular overlook in the park is Sunset Point, visited by 83% of park visitors, followed by Sunrise Point, visited by 76% of park visitors. It's an area near where Stephen Mather, a former director of the National Park Service, arrived when he first visited Bryce Canyon in 1919. A friend drove Mather to the rim and told him to keep his eyes closed until they arrived at the edge of it. When Mather opened his eyes, he gasped in wonder and promised to make Bryce Canyon a national park. In June 1923, President Warren G. Harding signed the bill to make Bryce Canyon a national monument—one of the last things he did in the White House. Departing on a trip through the western US, Harding visited Zion but not Bryce Canyon. A few weeks later, Harding died of a heart attack. Bryce became a national park in 1928.

The historic Bryce Canyon Lodge was designed by Yale-educated Gilbert Stanley Underwood, who also designed Zion Lodge, The Ahwahnee Hotel in Yosemite, and the Grand Canyon Lodge on the North Rim of the Grand Canyon—all classic examples of early National Park Service rustic

Rim Trail

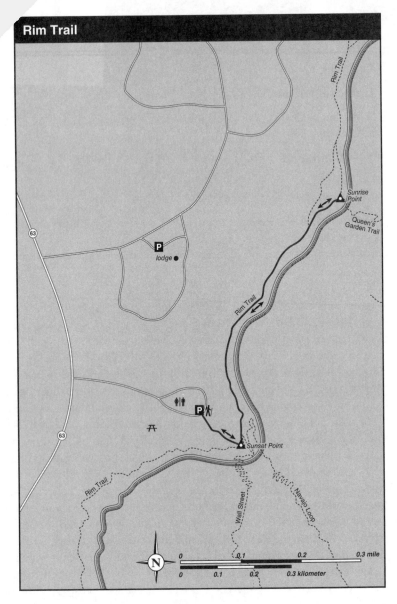

design. Built between 1924 and 1925 from locally quarried stones, including four monumental sandstone pillars reminiscent of the surrounding hoodoos, the lodge blends beautifully into the natural landscape of the Bryce Canyon rim. Of the national-park lodges designed by Underwood, Bryce Canyon Lodge is the only completely original structure still standing.

ROUTE

The Rim Trail is the route along the rim of Bryce Canyon from Fairyland Point (to the north) to Bryce Point (to the south). And while you can walk the entire 5.5-mile trail, you can cover more territory most efficiently by driving or taking the Bryce Canyon Shuttle to the various points and overlooks along the way, while doing most of your hiking on the more interesting below-the-rim trail through the Bryce Amphitheater and Fairyland. For that reason, what's included here is just the short paved section of the Rim Trail between Sunset Point and Sunrise Point.

It's a level, wide, and well-traveled route accessible to all—including wheelchair users and pets—and it's suitable for children, inexperienced hikers, and casual walkers.

The Sunset Point overlook gives you a view into the biggest natural amphitheater in the park. From Sunset Point walk along the paved path to Sunrise Point, a distance of only 0.5 mile. Here you can ascend the viewing platform and enjoy an equally splendid view of the Bryce Amphitheater from a more northerly perspective.

You can return to Sunset Point or board the Bryce Canyon Shuttle for your continued visit in the park.

TO THE TRAILHEAD
GPS Coordinates: N38º 12.573' W111º 10.145'
Drive 1.1 miles on UT 63 past the Bryce Canyon National Park entrance station to the Sunset Point turnoff, on the left. Then drive 0.2 mile to the Sunset Point parking area.

WHERE DO THOSE COLORS COME FROM?

While admiring the canyon, you'll observe rocks in a rainbow of colors. The reason for this multicolored spectacle is attributable to minerals in the rock. Hues of red, brown, black, or pink indicate that the rock contains the iron oxide mineral hematite. The yellow color comes from limonite, also an iron ore, and the lavender hues originate from the manganese dioxide pyrolusite. These minerals are mainly transported into the rock by groundwater. Dust-ingesting bacteria that live on the surface may also expel the minerals onto the rock.

15 Queens Garden and Navajo Loop

Trailhead Location: Sunrise Point, Bryce Canyon shuttle stop (*Note:* This hike can also be started from the Sunset Point parking area and shuttle stop.)

Trail Use: Walking, hiking

Distance & Configuration: 3.0-mile loop with various spurs and overlooks

Elevation Range: 8,015' at Sunrise Point to 7,400' in the wash near Queens Garden

Facilities: Restrooms, water, general store, and lodge near trailhead

Highlights: An exquisitely sculpted trail that goes into the heart of the hoodoos

DESCRIPTION

It would be easy to visit Bryce Canyon, drive the length of the park, stop at all the scenic turnoffs, and never stray more than 50 feet from your car, as thousands of visitors do each year. That would be a crying shame, though. To really experience Bryce, you need to dip below the rim and immerse yourself in the hoodoos. You need to experience the Bryce Amphitheater from inside the Bryce Amphitheater—not from a parking lot a mile away. Once you've descended below the rim, you're able to discover and explore the hoodoos, castles, and balanced rocks up close and from many angles.

Queens Garden and Navajo Loop is *the* signature hike in Bryce Canyon National Park. At the visitor center, rangers will regularly tell you that it's the best hike in the park. You may even see one of the interpretive signs in the visitor center touting it as the best 3-mile hike in America. Once again, there's no conceit in this claim. It would be difficult to find a better 3-mile hike anywhere in the world. Don't miss it.

Once you've committed to hiking to Queens Garden, you need to consider when to hike it. To beat the crowds, to avoid the scorching heat of the summer sun, and for the best photo conditions, hike the trail earlier in the day.

No hoodoo lasts forever. The formations and crumbly cliffs of Bryce Canyon are subject to rockfall, and nowhere is rockfall more prevalent than in the heart of the Bryce Amphitheater. Climbing on hoodoos is tempting,

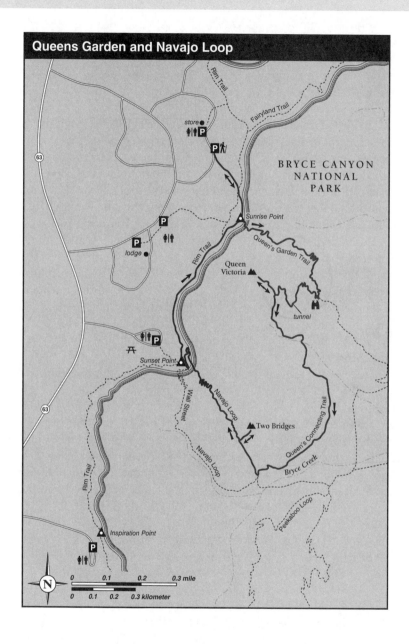

Queens Garden and Navajo Loop

Rim Trail

Fairyland Trail

store

P

BRYCE CANYON NATIONAL PARK

63

P

Sunrise Point

Queen's Garden Trail

lodge

Rim Trail

Queen Victoria

tunnel

Wall Street

Sunset Point

Navajo Loop

Two Bridges

Navajo Loop

Queen's Connecting Trail

Bryce Creek

63

Rim Trail

Peekaboo Loop

Inspiration Point

P

0   0.1   0.2   0.3 mile

0   0.1   0.2   0.3 kilometer

N

but those hand- and footholds are rated for chipmunks—nothing heavier. Rock climbing and scrambling on the gravelly slopes is illegal and dangerous, so stay on the trail and be aware of areas of potential rockfall.

ROUTE

From the parking area, stay on the paved trail for 0.1 mile before arriving at the rim and a sign pointing you in the direction of Queens Garden. Continue on this wide path for another 100 yards to reach Sunrise Point, where you'll begin your descent below the rim.

Initially the trail is wide, compacted, and well groomed, but it has steep drop-offs on both sides, so watch your step as you gaze at the astounding spread of formations below. At 0.5 mile from the trailhead, you'll come to a signed junction, with Queens Garden on the right and the horse trail to your left. Bear right and continue to Queens Garden. Then, in just another minute of walking, you arrive at a fork, where you'll make a hard right to stay on the trail (continuing straight ahead would have taken you to an overlook).

In another minute on the trail, you pass through a man-made tunnel as you descend into Queens Garden. Within the next few minutes, you'll pass through a second and third man-made tunnel, while the trail continues descending along tight switchbacks. As you exit the third tunnel, a spur trail on the right leads to the Queen Victoria hoodoo of Queens Garden. Within 100 yards you arrive at the base of the formation, which bears a striking resemblance to various statues in London of the monarch sitting on her throne.

Returning to the main trail, continue south in the direction of the Navajo Loop Trail. The trail cuts through a man-made divide between two hoodoos and enters a wash, where park visitors have been overly zealous in their placement of cairns. Passing through the wash, the trail veers south through the dappled shade of ponderosa pines before arriving at the junction with the Navajo Loop, where you begin your ascent to Sunset Point.

At 0.2 mile from the junction, you come to a short spur trail on the right that leads into a cathedral-like setting of hoodoos and the Two Bridges viewpoint. Leaving this area and returning to the main trail, the path becomes a ramp of 10 tightly carved and exquisitely sculpted switchbacks bound on both sides by hoodoos. Arriving at Sunset Point, you can complete the loop hike by making the short return to Sunrise Point on the level paved pathway.

TO THE TRAILHEAD

GPS Coordinates: N38º 12.573' W111º 10.145'

May–October, take the Bryce Canyon Shuttle to Sunrise Point. During other times of the year, enter the park on UT 63 and drive 0.4 mile past the Bryce Canyon National Park entrance to a signed road on the left, which leads to a picnic area and the North Campground. Bear right and follow the road to Bryce Canyon Lodge. After another 0.2 mile, turn left toward the general store; use the parking area marked for Sunrise Point.

HOW LONG DOES A HOODOO LAST?

The totem pole–shaped formations you see, known as hoodoos, are products of erosion. Formed in the various soft and hard layers of limestone and other types of sedimentary rock, their shapes are constantly changing. Experiencing more than 200 freeze–thaw cycles in a single year, hoodoos are frequently chipped away by expanding ice. The rainwater in the air is slightly acidic, which erodes the rock away grain by grain. Monsoons create heavy rainstorms and high winds that constantly bombard these rock formations. With an average erosional rate of 2–4 feet per 100 years, today's hoodoos will not always be there. They are constantly forming new cracks and holes that weaken them. The rock at Bryce Canyon is relatively soft; it erodes approximately 10–40% faster than the rock layers at Zion National Park. Even though the hoodoos' fate is inevitable, you can prevent premature erosion and help preserve them for future generations by staying on established trails.

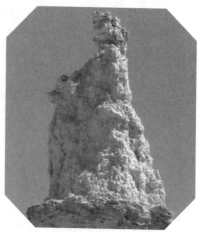

This Queens Garden hoodoo resembles a statue of Queen Victoria.

16 Tower Bridge

Trailhead Location: Sunrise Point, Bryce Canyon Shuttle Stop

Trail Use: Walking, hiking

Distance & Configuration: 4.0-mile out-and-back

Elevation Range: 8,015' at Sunrise Point to 7,150' at the base of Tower Bridge

Facilities: Restrooms, water, general store, and lodge near trailhead

Highlights: Classic Bryce Canyon scenery and formations in a less-visited section of the park

DESCRIPTION

This out-and-back from Sunrise Point to Tower Bridge, on the southern side of the Fairyland Loop, is a great option for those who want the off-the-beaten-track experience of the Fairyland Loop but lack the time required to hike the entire route. With this hike comes some of the best scenery of the loop in about half the distance—a fair trade, most would agree.

The trail's namesake formation, Tower Bridge, is not really a natural bridge but an arch. The name is derived from the hoodoo's similarity to Tower Bridge, the twin-towered suspension bridge near the Tower of London in the UK.

The Tower Bridge Trail offers moderate hiking, with 865 feet of elevation descent and gain in the span of around 3 miles. So it's a good workout that's still well suited for families and less-experienced hikers.

ROUTE

Starting at the familiar and popular Sunrise Point shuttle stop, follow the marked Rim Trail to the north, away from Sunrise Point and in the direction of Fairyland Loop. Arriving at the junction of the Tower Bridge Trail, turn right and descend through bristlecone pines and brightly colored gullies. As you descend the Tower Bridge Trail, you'll see sections of the Chinese Wall on your right and Campbell Canyon on the left.

Reaching the bottom of the canyon, at about 1.5 miles from the Tower Bridge Trail junction, you'll see a trail sign directing you on and to the left for a continuation to the Fairyland Loop—instead, take the short spur descending to your right in the marked direction of Tower Bridge. This

Tower Bridge

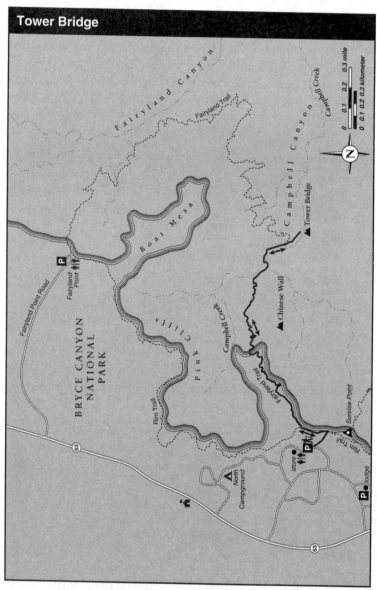

leads to a comfy and shaded lunch spot that's the perfect location for viewing Tower Bridge. The fin capped by Tower Bridge is also home to Keyhole Window, another captivating formation set on the same geologic layer and to the left of Tower Bridge. Soak in the view and rest in the shade before beginning your upward trek back to the rim the way you came.

TO THE TRAILHEAD

GPS Coordinates: N38° 12.573' W111° 10.145'

May–October, take the Bryce Canyon Shuttle to Sunrise Point. During other times of the year, enter Bryce Canyon National Park on UT 63. Drive 0.4 mile past the park entrance to a signed road on the left that leads to a picnic area and the North Campground. Bear right and follow the road to Bryce Canyon Lodge. After another 0.2 mile, turn left toward the general store; use the parking area marked for Sunrise Point.

IS IT AN ARCH OR A BRIDGE?

Distinguishing between an arch and a bridge can be confusing. The following definitions will help you decide which formation you are viewing. On a natural arch, the frame is intact, and a hole has formed completely through it. The rock is surrounded by air and completely exposed to the elements. It has been formed by natural erosion processes (such as wind and water). A natural bridge is a type of arch where a water current, such as a stream, carved the hole; in some cases the water still flows through the opening.

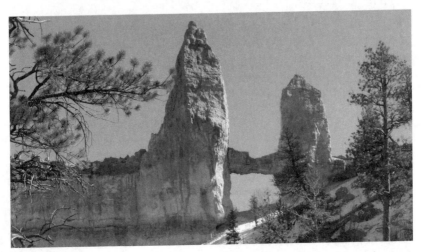

Tower Bridge

17 Fairyland Loop

Trailhead Location: Fairyland Point

Trail Use: Walking, hiking

Distance & Configuration: 8.2-mile loop

Elevation Range: 7,787' at trailhead to 7,142' in Fairyland Canyon and 8,075' on the Pink Cliffs near the rim

Facilities: None

Highlights: A less-crowded trail plunging deep into Bryce Canyon wilderness with varied views

DESCRIPTION

Bryce Canyon is relatively compact as national parks go, so finding an off-the-beaten route not already lined with tourists shortly after sunrise may seem unachievable. But that's what you'll find in Fairyland, a lesser-known bowl on the park's northern fringe. You will actually access the trailhead and hike in Fairyland before ever entering the park.

Fairyland is in an earlier stage of formation than the more mature Bryce Amphitheater. As a result, the landscape provides a smaller and more intimate experience than the immense bowls and well-known amphitheaters farther south in the park. Granted, the scenery in Fairyland isn't as dramatic or awe-inspiring as what you'll find in the Bryce Amphitheater, but it still holds a number of noteworthy formations and great hiking. While Fairyland may not be on anyone's must-do list in Bryce, it certainly is worthy of your time on a second or third day in the park, after you've seen the more popular bowls. Like many other areas in the park, it's best photographed at sunrise.

Because Fairyland is a younger formation, the effects of storms and erosion are more instantly noticeable here. With each rainstorm or the melting of snowpack, the water washes sand and pebbles away toward the Paria River, and it's easier to imagine that the ground you're walking on will someday be a hoodoo standing tall and proud.

ROUTE

Your adventure in Fairyland will normally begin at the Fairyland Loop trailhead, as described here, though you can also access the area from Sunrise

Fairyland Loop

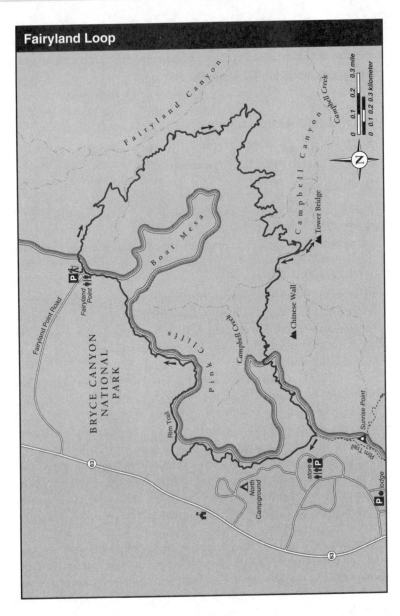

Point, on the southwest side of the loop. (And in winter, when the road to Fairyland Point is closed, the only way to hike it is from Sunrise Point.) Soon after leaving the trailhead, you enter the Bryce Canyon Wilderness Area—the backcountry of the canyon.

The trail descends into Fairyland Canyon with small arches and a variety of hoodoos popping into view; Boat Mesa, a prominent, 8,076-foot-high plateau, rises in the near distance on the right. Fairyland Loop circumnavigates this mesa. The hike consists of dozens of switchbacks and hairpin turns, which take you bobbing and weaving your way around the myriad formations, finger canyons, and small draws—all in the presence of ponderosa pines, Utah junipers, and manzanitas.

After descending into the bottom of the wash in Fairyland Canyon, the trail steadily ascends several switchbacks to attain an overview to the east. This overlook is easily accessed on an unmarked spur about 100 feet off the main trail to the left. Beyond the spur, you'll ascend for about 100 yards to witness another sweeping overlook to the south.

After 4.0 miles from the trailhead you'll arrive at the best-known and most-identifiable natural formation on the Fairyland Loop: Tower Bridge, which bears an uncanny similarity to its Thames-spanning namesake in London. You'll obtain the best view of Tower Bridge from a short spur on the left, marked by a sign.

Departing Tower Bridge the trail makes a steady and not-too-demanding ascent back to the Rim Trail in 1.7 miles. By bearing right and proceeding north across the gentle undulations of the Pink Cliffs, you'll return to the Fairyland Point trailhead and parking area, on your left in 2.5 miles, to complete the loop.

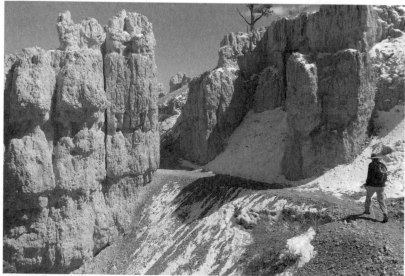
Fairyland Loop

TO THE TRAILHEAD

GPS Coordinates: N37° 38.968' W112° 8.843'

From the junction of UT 12 and UT 63, proceed south on UT 63 for 3 miles to signed Fairyland Point Road on the left, 0.8 mile before you arrive at the park entrance station and visitor center. Continue on Fairyland Point Road for 1.0 mile to the viewpoint parking area.

GREENLEAF MANZANITA

Characterized by smooth, leathery, reddish bark, this evergreen shrub grows throughout Bryce Canyon National Park. If you're hiking in the spring, you may have the opportunity to see its beautiful pink flowers. The greenleaf manzanita holds its leaves vertically, in contrast to other plants that hold their

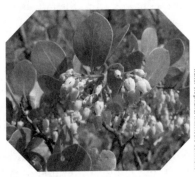

leaves horizontally. This reduces sun exposure and prevents heavy snow from weighing the shrub down. Reportedly, a Bryce park ranger offered to pay visitors $1 for every horizontal manzanita leaf they found—a bet he never had to pay out.

Throughout history, the manzanita shrub has had many uses. Its berries have provided food as well as natural remedies and antiseptics. Today, many people plant manzanita trees for decorative or landscape use. While hiking in Utah's national parks, be aware that manzanita trees are protected so they can be enjoyed by all.

18 Water Canyon and Moss

Trailhead Location: A small parking area on th
UT 12, just 3.7 miles east of its junction with UT

Trail Use: Walking, hiking

Distance & Configuration: 1.0-mile out-and-back, including
a short spur to Mossy Cave

Elevation Range: 6,840' at trailhead to 6,950' at Mossy Cave

Facilities: Vault toilets at trailhead

Highlights: Wet, often ice-filled cave and nearby waterfall

DESCRIPTION

The presence of water in Water Canyon is a tribute to the early settlers who
dug a 10-mile irrigation canal by hand in 1892 to bring water from the
East Fork Sevier River to the Paria Valley. The canal was successful in sus-
taining desert farming communities and also created a scenic canyon with
a stream—the only stream in Bryce Canyon National Park.

The cave, cooling stream, and waterfall make this a fun short hike
that's well suited to hikers of all ages and abilities. The location on UT 12,
in the northern section of the park just east of the park entrance, makes
Water Canyon a convenient place to stop and stretch your legs after several
hours in the car and before entering the heart of Bryce Canyon.

ROUTE

From the roadside parking area, the wide trail ascends gently into the canyon amid hoodoos on the upper slopes that cast a glow of orange and white.
Although Water Canyon is not large, it has a sense of openness, with a mix
of bristlecone and limber pines on the surrounding slopes.

You'll appreciate the sturdy bridge with the metal railing. The two
bridges are fairly recent additions and replace numerous previous bridges that
had been washed away during flash floods. It's hard to imagine that the small
stream you're crossing could swell to a torrent capable of washing out a bridge,
but it gives you a sense of the potential for flash flooding in a desert canyon.

The canal that brings the stream into Water Canyon has a rather inglo-
rious name—Tropic Ditch—but a proud history. The stream has been in
existence just over 100 years, but it has already had a profound effect on
the canyon ecosystem, attracting wildlife not previously seen in the area.

Water Canyon and Mossy Cave

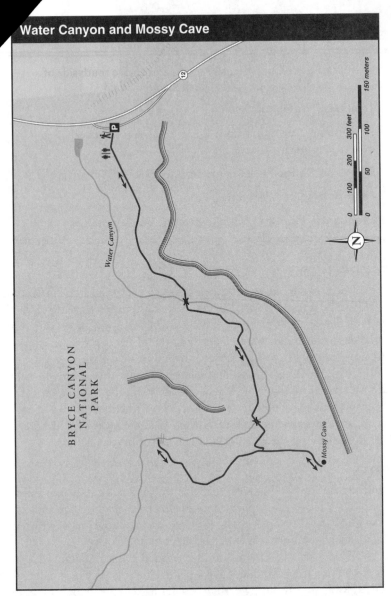

Flora such as the Watson bog orchid and the mountain deathcamas appear in the now-watered canyon, and over time the geology of the canyon will continue to become more like other V-shaped stream-cut canyons.

After crossing the bridge, the trail ascends more steeply and soon arrives at a fork. Take the route to the left that leads on to Mossy Cave. Technically more a grotto or alcove than a cave, Mossy Cave invites inspection nonetheless. This shallow, moss-filled alcove, fed by an underground spring, is adorned with ferns and, in winter, icicles.

Now returning down the trail to the fork, take the branch to the right (north) this time to head in the direction of the waterfall. This 15-foot plunge drops into a circular pool exposing dolomite limestone bedrock. The pools are perfect for a refreshing break on a hot summer day.

Along with the hoodoos, you can also spot several windows sculpted into the rock above the falls to your right. A short trail leads to the window and makes for a fun add-on with some great views down to the waterfall. Retrace your route down the canyon to return to the trailhead.

TO THE TRAILHEAD

GPS Coordinates: N37º 39.946' W112º 6.619'

From the junction of UT 63 and UT 12, continue east on UT 12 for 3.7 miles to a small parking area on the south side of the highway.

TROPIC DITCH

In 1874 a few pioneers heard about the Paria Valley from American Indians. It sounded appealing, with a favorable climate, abundant grazing, arable land, timber, coal, and water. The pioneers soon settled the communities of Cannonville and Henrieville, which lie to the east of Bryce Canyon on the Paria River.

But the growth of these communities forced farmers to look for more reliable water sources than the seasonal flow of the Paria River. They conceived a plan to bring water from the East Fork Sevier River on the Paunsaugunt Plateau to the west of Bryce Canyon to augment the flow of the Paria.

From 1890 to 1892, Mormon pioneers labored with picks and shovels to carve a 10-mile canal across the Paunsaugunt Plateau. Since that time, except during the drought of 2002, Tropic Ditch has supplied irrigation water to the Paria Valley. The water rights extend from mid-April to mid-October, when you'll see water pouring over the falls and down the canyon.

Canyonlands National Park

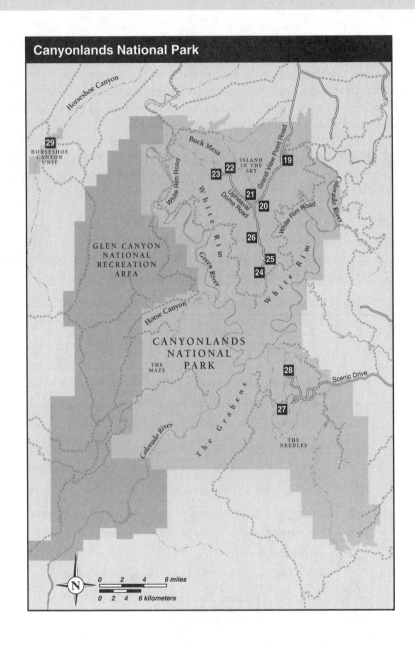

CANYONLANDS NATIONAL PARK

Park Overview

Canyonlands, Utah's largest national park, is an immense wilderness of mesas, buttes, sandstone fins, spires, and canyons—hundreds of them—carved by the Colorado River, the Green River, and their tributaries. Canyonlands is also Utah's least-visited national park, and one that's difficult to visit in a day or two because it's divided into four districts: Island in the Sky, The Needles, The Maze, and the rivers themselves. No bridges or roads connect one district to another, so travel between them takes hours by car.

When the park was established in 1964, the land was known to just a small number of ranchers and miners. Even today, it's a remote, untamed wilderness with few paved roads, not many power lines, and precious little piped water. It remains one of the last relatively undisturbed regions of the Colorado Plateau.

With fewer than 10 inches of rainfall per year and elevations ranging from 3,700 to 7,200 feet above sea level, Canyonlands is high desert, so expect hot summers, cold winters, and the potential for surprises, such as flash floods and temperatures that can fluctuate as much as 50°F over the course of 24 hours.

JUST ONE DAY?

Given the park's size, remoteness, and lack of connecting roads, it's best to limit your visit to just one district. If you plan on combining the trip with one to neighboring Arches National Park, Island in the Sky would be an excellent choice. Starting at the Island in the Sky Visitor Center, continue on to Mesa Arch, then on to Grand View Point, each with short hikes and panoramic views. For some elevation gain and fun red-rock hiking, you'll enjoy Aztec Butte, with the short Crater View Trail as your concluding hike for the day.

If your travels take you south of Moab, then The Needles district is a great place to explore. Elephant Hill to Chesler Park (page 116) is one of the finest hikes in Utah.

◘ ◘ ◘

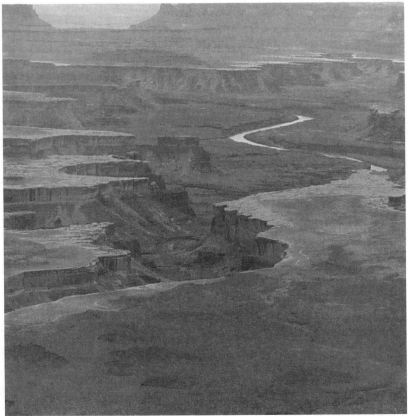

Spectacular vistas on the Grand View Point Trail (see Hike 24, page 107)

19 Neck Spring Loop Trail

Trailhead Location: Neck Spring Parking Area in the Island in the Sky district

Trail Use: Walking, hiking

Distance & Configuration: 5.8-mile loop

Elevation Range: 6,450' at trailhead to 6,150' at the springs level below the rim

Facilities: None

Highlights: Pure spring water flows from a desert cliff, creating a microhabitat.

DESCRIPTION

The Neck Spring Loop Trail is the best of the very few loops within the Island in the Sky district, a labyrinthine plateau where most of the trails are out-and-backs or connectors. But here we follow a counterclockwise route that takes us below the rim and brings us back up to the plateau on the return to our starting point.

The Neck is an unusual topographic feature: a 40-foot-wide land bridge with sheer drop-offs and gaping canyons on both sides. As such, this narrow strip of land offers the only vehicle access to the Island in the Sky.

The Neck also has historical significance, as American Indians may have set brush traps or fences across it to capture bighorn sheep or other game. Later, ranchers used this area as a natural gate with which they could corral livestock on the Island. Putting up and maintaining fences was time-consuming work for ranchers, and here they could manage the entire 43-square-mile mesa with just one 40-foot fence.

On this parched plateau of the desert Southwest, perennial sources of water were essential for any type of settlement. So the trickles of both Neck Spring and Cabin Spring were vital water sources for nearby commercial livestock operations in the early 20th century. The rusted and broken troughs and other apparatus are another reminder of the challenges early settlers faced in this harsh desert environment.

ROUTE

The Neck Spring Loop Trail begins on the southwest side of the parking area, where a sign marks the start of the trail. You'll make a short drop

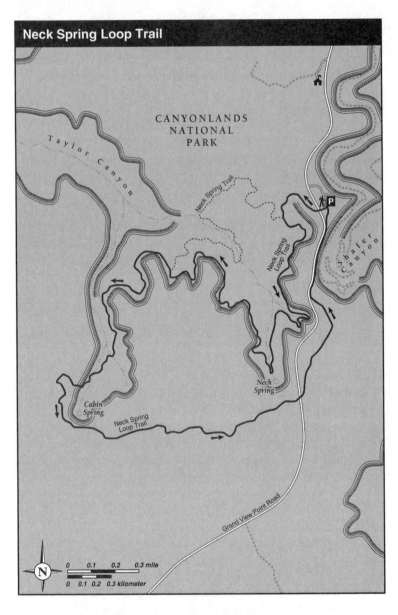

Neck Spring Loop Trail

from the parking lot, cross the road, and begin your descent into the canyon to start the counterclockwise loop. As you descend, the color of the trail changes from a whitish upper layer of Navajo Sandstone into the more characteristic red cliff layers of the same formation. It's often windy on top of the plateau, but once you drop below the rim, you'll find some calming protection from the elements.

As you drop below the canyon rim and pass the Neck Spring Trail cut-off on your right, the trail stays on a fairly level contour and hugs the canyon wall on your left. About 20 minutes from the trailhead, you approach an alcove on the canyon wall, where the undercut cliff rises 200 feet above. This alcove and others like it are created when a softer formation erodes and creates an overhang below a harder formation. You'll see very minor seepage but no water flow. At this point, make a hairpin turn and continue on the trail, exiting the alcove.

The trail soon rounds the bend to enter a similarly formed side canyon. It again approaches the head of an alcove, but this time you'll find a bit more water as you step across the flow without ever wetting the soles of your shoes. This is Neck Spring, on the north side of The Neck. Neck Spring is just a trickle—by modern standards little more than a leaky faucet—but this would have been enough water flow to induce pioneers to settle here.

As you pass though Neck Spring, observe the microhabitat that the water creates. You'll find species in this alcove that exist nowhere else on the nearby plateau, including Gambel oaks, small Fremont cottonwoods, and maidenhair ferns. As you can see, it doesn't take very much water to create such a distinctive microhabitat.

Leaving Neck Spring, the trail undulates, but it stays at the same general level in the canyon, contouring along with the twists and turns carved by water and erosion. The path enters several sequential dry canyons,

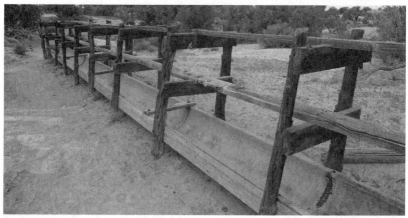

Remains of a water trough on Neck Spring Trail

similar in shape and formation to Neck Spring alcove but without the life-sustaining water.

In another 5 minutes beyond Neck Spring, you come to a second spring, again not much more than a trickle and barely visible in its flow. This is Cabin Spring. Immediately after you pass Cabin Spring, the trail rises up from the canyon on a steep, short ascent along slickrock marked by cairns.

Within minutes you're back up above the rim on a trail that winds through desert brush interspersed by stretches of slickrock. Arriving at an old weather-beaten trough, the route veers left and continues across the plateau overviews of Taylor Canyon, its alcoves, and trail below.

Soon the trail crosses the road to complete the loop and return you to the Neck Spring Parking Area. As the parking area comes into view, about 0.5 mile away, the trail parallels the road on your left to bring you safely back to your car.

TO THE TRAILHEAD

GPS Coordinates: N38º 27.143' W109º 49.227'
Drive 0.5 mile south of the Island in the Sky Visitor Center on Grand View Point Road to the Neck Spring Parking Area, on the left.

NATURAL SPRINGS IN THE DESERT

Water is scarce in the high desert and essential to the native ecology in the area. During the drier times of year, the natural springs are critical to wildlife that are unable to travel long distances to rivers. At these springs, you'll see a high concentration of flora and fauna, with some of those species clustered in microhabitats. Many of the plants and animals would be unable to survive if these vital water sources didn't exist. Small actions from hikers, such as taking a swim while covered in sunscreen or throwing garbage into the water, can pollute these resources. While visiting the springs, make sure to cause as little impact on them as possible—the lives of the desert's inhabitants depend on it.

20 Mesa Arch Loop

Trailhead Location: Mesa Arch Parking Area in the Island in the Sky district

Trail Use: Walking, hiking

Distance & Configuration: 0.8-mile balloon

Elevation Range: 6,155' at trailhead to 6,123' at Mesa Arch

Facilities: None

Highlights: A short, popular hike with something for everyone, including an arch perched right on the rim at the end

DESCRIPTION

It's a quick jaunt to Mesa Arch, the most scenic and accessible stone arch in Canyonlands. This hike is suitable for all ages and skill levels and highly recommended for every park visitor. It's a great way to start your day in Island in the Sky after first stopping at the visitor center.

Mesa Arch is a Navajo Sandstone arch made especially photogenic by its setting on the edge of a 500-foot cliff. It perfectly frames the La Sal Mountains in the distance and Buck Canyon 1,200 feet below. You'll also have views of Washer Woman Arch from the overlook.

ROUTE

The trailhead parking area lies on the fringe of Gray's Pasture, where you'll have views of Aztec Butte to the west and the Henry Mountains to the southwest, nearly 60 miles in the distance. Signs at the trailhead identify plants along the trail—plants that you'll seeing throughout your visit to Canyonlands and the other national parks in Utah. In addition, small signs on the ground identify many of the native shrubs and trees. Knowing just a handful of these plants will enhance your visit. Some of these familiar native species include Mormon tea (ephedra), blackbrush, littleleaf mountain-mahogany, and prickly pear cactus. Just beyond the interpretive signs, a wide and well-compacted stairway leads to the top of a small knoll.

The trail is so wide and well defined that most visitors miss the branch of the path veering to the left, which forms the loop. If you're one of them, don't worry, as you'll still arrive safely at Mesa Arch, although the return is more difficult to find once you're at the arch.

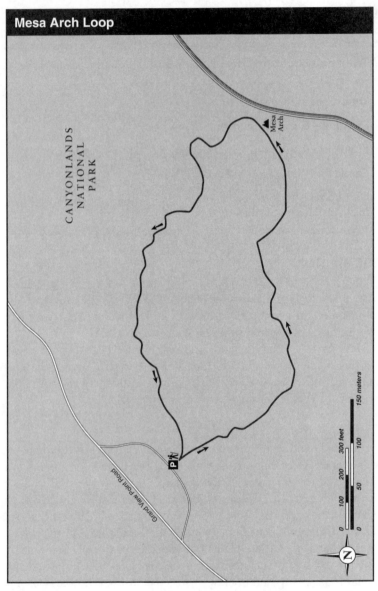

Just beyond the wide steps, the path curves to the left and flattens before arriving at Mesa Arch. The arch invites play, as you'll want to climb onto its face, sheltered by its span. With Mesa Arch as a frame and the snowcapped La Sal Mountains as the backdrop, even a rank amateur can become an artistic portrait photographer. Below the horizon you'll gaze into the depths

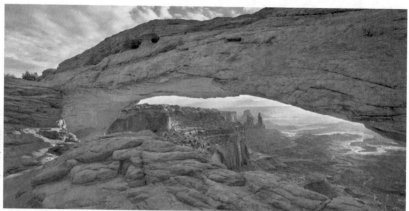

Mesa Arch

of Buck Canyon, sculpted by the Colorado River. You can return to the trailhead by completing the loop or returning the way you came.

TO THE TRAILHEAD

GPS Coordinates: N38º 23.346' W109º 52.080'
Drive 6.1 miles south of the Island in the Sky Visitor Center on Grand View Point Road, and turn left into the Mesa Arch Parking Area.

DEAD HORSE POINT

The dramatic overlook and its evocative name have a story behind them. In the 19th century, local cowboys used a natural corral at Dead Horse Point to hold wild horses that were rounded up in the area. The only way out of the corral was a fenced-off 30-yard opening. When the corral was abandoned, the gate to the corral was left open so the horses could return to the open range. Unfortunately, none of the horses left, staying in the enclosure until they met their demise. Today, Dead Horse Point is a Utah state park featuring spectacular viewpoints and interpretive displays about the area's natural history. You'll pass the entrance to the state park before arriving at the Canyonlands National Park entrance.

21 Aztec Butte Trail

Trailhead Location: Aztec Butte Trailhead, Island in the Sky district

Trail Use: Walking, hiking

Distance & Configuration: 2.5-mile balloon with spur

Elevation Range: 6,098' at trailhead to 6,310' on top of Aztec Butte

Facilities: None

Highlights: An adventurous hike to an ancestral Puebloan granary and structures with commanding views

DESCRIPTION

From high above the mesa, one of the highest elevations in Canyonlands, Aztec Butte overlooks sheer cliffs and labyrinthine canyons in every direction. As you scramble up these steep slickrock faces in high-traction trail shoes and ultralight day packs, consider the ancestral Puebloans shod in yucca sandals and laden with baskets of grain as they ascended these buttes to store their harvest in small stone structures sealed with mud. These beautifully preserved granaries still stand today as a testament to the ingenuity and determination of people who survived in this desert climate.

The climb to the top of Aztec Butte—not for the fainthearted—traverses steep slopes and uneven terrain, with precipitous drop-offs, and requires mounting and descending ledges up to 3 feet high. Some scrambling on

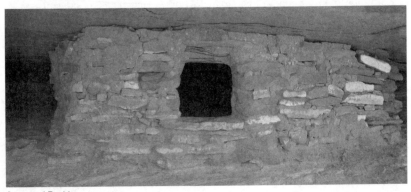

Ancestral Puebloan granary

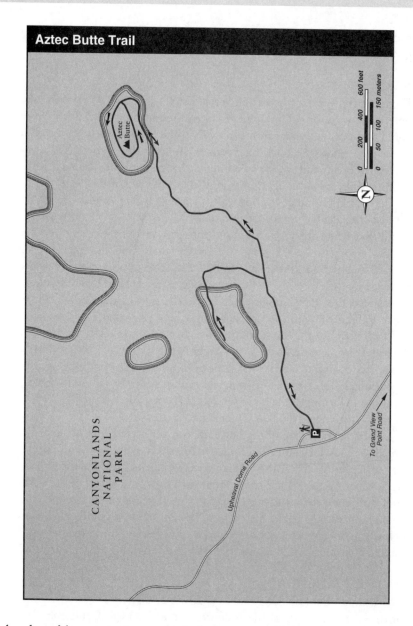

hands and knees may be required. A short spur off the main trail ascends the lower butte to two small granaries.

One final reminder: Climbing on or tampering with archeological sites is strictly prohibited. That these magnificent granaries remain standing today is miraculous. Let's do everything we can to preserve them for future generations.

ROUTE

From the trailhead at the parking area, you'll make a slight descent before entering a wash of golden sand on an eastbound trail. At 0.3 mile, you'll come to a trail junction marked only by a cairn and a particularly vibrant piñon tree—take the trail that veers to the left. This spur makes a quick and not-too-difficult ascent, climbing slickrock onto the butte on the left. Within 100 yards from the junction, you'll be on top of the butte.

Crossing the top of the butte for 0.1 mile, you arrive at the north edge of the butte, at which point the trail makes a small dip below the edge. Here you'll easily find the granary tucked into an alcove beneath a small overhang. As you admire the granary, consider what it took for ancient people more than a thousand years ago to find a suitable location perennially protected from the elements, and then to build a granary and haul water to mix the cement to seal the granary. Complete the spur by descending this first butte and returning to the junction from which you came.

Once back at the junction, turn left and continue across the desert for another 0.1 mile to the base of the larger of the two buttes. What starts out as an easy ascent up a slickrock slope becomes very steep, though passable if you follow the cairns and switchback your way up the face of the butte. It takes a sure footing and a bit of scrambling, especially on the last 30 feet of ascent, but soon you'll be on top of Aztec Butte.

Once you're on top of the butte, mark your arrival spot by identifying a plant or rock formation you'll recognize as you complete your clockwise loop of the butte's top. The trail makes a 0.2-mile loop around the top of the mesa, where on the far side of the loop you'll discover the remains of a structure. This time the structure comprises the remains of stone walls, likely from an ancestral Puebloan structure, though not necessarily a habitation. When you've completed the loop, make your descent at the spot where you marked your ascent, and return to the trailhead parking area.

TO THE TRAILHEAD

GPS Coordinates: N38° 23.609' W109° 52.914'

Drive 6.3 miles south of the Island in the Sky Visitor Center on Grand View Point Road, and turn right at the junction onto Upheaval Dome Road. Continue 0.9 mile to the Aztec Butte Parking Area, on the right.

GRANARIES

Aztec Butte is a misnomer; the ancient people who lived in the Canyonlands area and built the granaries here weren't Aztecs, but rather Anasazi, also known as ancestral Puebloans. The granaries, which date back as far as AD 1200–1300, were built in protected plateau areas and were mainly used as storage facilities. The American Indians resided closer to water sources and would climb up to the plateau to store collected food, including maize, beans, and squash. These granaries represented a lot of hard work and ingenuity on the part of the region's ancient inhabitants. They were placed in areas where they would be protected from flooding or moisture from rainfall (high on cliffs and under overhangs). The storage places were also sealed with mud to prevent desert critters from getting in and eating an entire year's store of grain. Considerable work was involved in carrying the grain to these storehouses, and also in transporting water, often for several miles, to make the mud. These granaries were widely used until weather patterns changed, making growing crops difficult. The Anasazi eventually moved farther south, toward New Mexico and Arizona, where some of their descendants live today.

22 Whale Rock Trail

Trailhead Location: Whale Rock Trailhead in the Island in the Sky district

Trail Use: Walking, hiking

Distance & Configuration: 1.0-mile out-and-back

Elevation Range: 5,719' at Whale Rock Trailhead to 5,863' at the crest of Whale Rock

Facilities: None

Highlights: Short climb to the top of a whale-shaped slickrock dome

DESCRIPTION

Whale Rock is a great short hike that delivers a 360-degree panoramic overview of the entire Island in the Sky region. As you drive down Upheaval Dome Road, Whale Rock is easy to spot—it's the rock that looks like a whale. Is it a blue whale or a beluga? You decide. You can be sure of one thing, though: This is a fun romp for families and kids of all ages.

The first section of the trail passes through sand and over outcrops of slickrock to the top. Then, as you ascend the rock, the trail is set entirely on

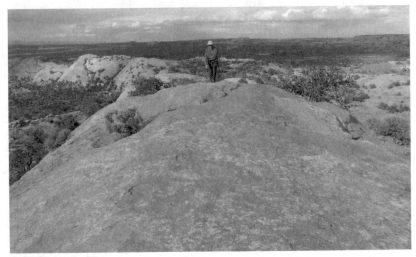

Whale Rock summit

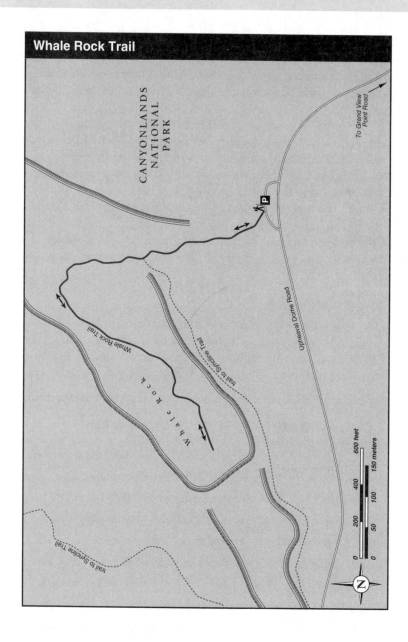

Whale Rock Trail

CANYONLANDS NATIONAL PARK

To Grand View Point Road

Upheaval Dome Road

Whale Rock Trail

trail to Syncline Trail

Whale Rock

trail to Syncline Trail

600 feet
400
200
0

150 meters
100
50
0

N

slickrock. You'll see the patches in the slickrock surface to cover the holes
that once supported stanchions and cables, now removed to give the park
a more natural face, but the cemented cairns remain.

ROUTE

From the trailhead parking area, a gravel path takes off to the north and soon begins to contour along the edge of a slickrock slope. Mounting the slope, gently at first and then steepening, you'll soon find yourself climbing the whale's back from the tail to the head.

At 0.3 mile you're on top of this beautifully rounded slickrock dome. Continuing on, you come to the highest point on Whale Rock, at about 0.4 mile. You can continue forward, but you'll eventually come to a point approaching the whale's head where the slope is too steep to permit onward travel, so stopping at the crest is probably your best bet.

From the crest of the whale, you'll have views to the north as far as the San Rafael Swell. One view you won't have is the Upheaval Dome, which is nearby and actually part of the same formation as Whale Rock. From the unshaded crest, you can enjoy the views and then make your return to the trailhead.

TO THE TRAILHEAD

GPS Coordinates: N38º 25.613' W109º 54.842'
Drive 6.3 miles south of the Island in the Sky Visitor Center on Grand View Point Road, and turn right at the junction onto Upheaval Dome Road. Continue 3.9 miles to the Whale Rock Parking Area, on the right.

IT'S NOT A CROW; IT'S A RAVEN!

These intelligent local residents can be found year-round in the state of Utah. Ravens grow up to 24 inches tall with a wingspan of more than 4 feet, and with their distinguishing call, they are hard to miss. Ravens are scavengers and will eat just about anything. Besides eating leftovers, they are known to eat berries and hunt for small bugs, reptiles, and rodents. They build bulky stick nests in shady locations that have a good platform. While hiking in Utah, you have a good chance of seeing one of these beautiful birds.

---

23 Crater View Trail and Upheaval Dome Overlook

Trailhead Location: Upheaval Dome Picnic Area in the Island in the Sky district

Trail Use: Walking, hiking

Distance & Configuration: 1.8-mile out-and-back

Elevation Range: 5,705' at trailhead to 5,855' at overlook

Facilities: Vault toilets, shaded picnic tables, and fire grates at trailhead

Highlights: Short hike across slickrock to an overview of an unexplained dimple deep in the canyon

DESCRIPTION

Crater View Trail, a short, steeply pitched trail, leads to a dramatic overlook on the south rim of Upheaval Dome and returns along the same route, with an elevation gain of 200 feet. The attraction here is Upheaval Dome, a geologic oddity and somewhat of an unsolved mystery. Is it an

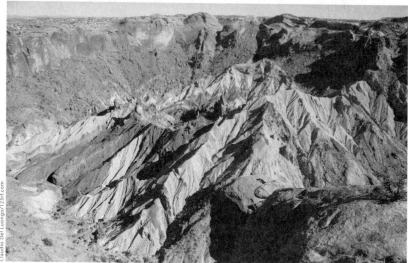

Claudio Del Luongo/123rf.com

View of Upheaval Dome from the rim

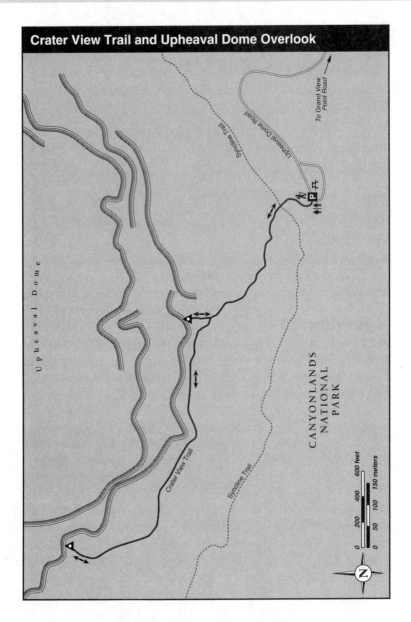

Crater View Trail and Upheaval Dome Overlook

upward flowing mass of salt or a meteor crater? Because scientists may never solve the mystery of what it is and how it formed, you might as well go see for yourself and add your two cents to the debate. You just may be right.

In addition to the fame and stature you'll receive in the scientific community if you're correct, you'll also have some great views over an expanse of mesas and a maze of canyons that gives Canyonlands its name. The air quality in southern Utah gives Canyonlands and Capitol Reef some of the longest views in North America, so it wouldn't be uncommon for your gaze on one of these overlooks to encompass more than 1,000 square miles. The appearance of clouds, rain, or lightning marching across the horizon in the far distance only makes the scenery more exciting.

ROUTE

From the parking area, the trail rises steadily and steeply on a well-crafted route reinforced with sandstone blocks and surrounded by jumbled Kayenta Formation blocks and stone. Because you're near a picnic area, you're also likely to see ravens and piñon jays, both smart birds and capable of waiting until you turn your back or walk away from the table before flying off with your snacks or lunches.

At 85 yards you'll come to a four-way junction with the Syncline Loop Trail, one of the most strenuous trails in the park and one that descends below the rim to make a loop around the Upheaval Dome. Continue straight in the signed direction of the overlook. Continuing your climb on slickrock outcrops of Kayenta Formation ledges, you arrive in 0.2 mile from the trailhead at a sign directing you to a short spur on the right, where in 50 yards you arrive at the first overlook. Here you'll find an interpretive display that explains the theories on the origins of Upheaval Dome. At this overlook you have some fine vistas stretching to the north, as well as an excellent bird's-eye view of Upheaval Dome below.

Returning to the main trail, turn right at the junction and continue to the second overlook, another 0.7 mile along the trail to the west. The path to the second overlook undulates along cairned slickrock before arriving at the fenced overlook. If you know what you're looking for, or if you have a larger area map in hand, you'll recognize features in the distance to the southwest and north, including the Henry Mountains, the San Rafael Reef, and the Book Cliffs.

Return to the parking area the way you came. As long as you're on Upheaval Dome Road, on your way back to the visitor center via your car, don't miss one of the great overviews in the park: the Green River Overview. Before reaching the visitor center, turn right at the sign in the direction of Green River Overview, and drive to the end of the 1.5-mile road. The overview is at the parking area, and no real hiking is required.

TO THE TRAILHEAD

GPS Coordinates: N38º 25.579' W109º 55.564'

Drive 6.3 miles south of the Island in the Sky Visitor Center on Grand View Point Road and turn right at the junction onto Upheaval Dome Road. Continue 5.1 miles to the Upheaval Dome Picnic Area loop, at the end of the road.

UPHEAVAL DOME

Upheaval Dome, which you'll see from the Crater View Trail, is a fascinating geologic feature unlike anything else nearby. The mystery of how this large circular depression formed remains unsolved. One theory suggests that an upward flowing mass of salt formed it. The overlaying rock from above was denser than the salt, causing the salt to slowly float to the surface like a bubble. The salt eroded, leaving only the harder rock layers behind. Another theory suggests that the feature was formed 600 million years ago when a large meteor roughly 0.3 mile in diameter struck the area, providing a pathway for the salt to move toward the surface. One puzzling feature: Upheaval Dome contains surface rock that can only be found a mile or more underground anywhere else in the surrounding area.

---

24 Grand View Point Trail

Trailhead Location: Grand View Point Parking Area in the Island in the Sky district

Trail Use: Walking, hiking

Distance & Configuration: 2.0-mile out-and-back

Elevation Range: 6,266' at trailhead to 6,226' at tip of Grand View Point

Facilities: Vault toilets at trailhead; no water

Highlights: An aptly named trail follows a cliffside route to a dramatic conclusion.

DESCRIPTION

Grand View Point is the best of three similar overview hikes on the Grand View Mesa; the other two are Murphy Point and the White Rim Overlook. If you only do one of these hikes, make it the Grand View Point Trail—it delivers the most impressive and panoramic view of the Canyonlands basin in the entire park.

The trail sticks close to the canyon rim throughout, never departing more than about 20 feet from sheer cliff at any point. Along the way you'll traverse the Kayenta Formation, resting solidly on a base of Wingate Sandstone.

As you work out the details of your visit to the Island in the Sky, Grand View, located at the farthest extension of the paved park road, can be conveniently and efficiently hiked at any point in the day—first thing in the morning, at midday, or at sunset—and while your experience will likely be different as the light catches the canyon at different angles, it will always be rewarding.

ROUTE

Not only is Grand View the best overlook hike in the park, but because it's a popular overview, it has some of the best interpretive signage of any trail in the Island in the Sky. You'll see many of these interpretive signs in the parking area and at the Grand View Overlook, on a wheelchair-accessible paved route just a hundred feet from the parking area.

From the overlook, the Grand View Point Trail departs from the wheelchair-accessible paved lookout to the southwest, with steep drop-offs

Grand View Point Trail

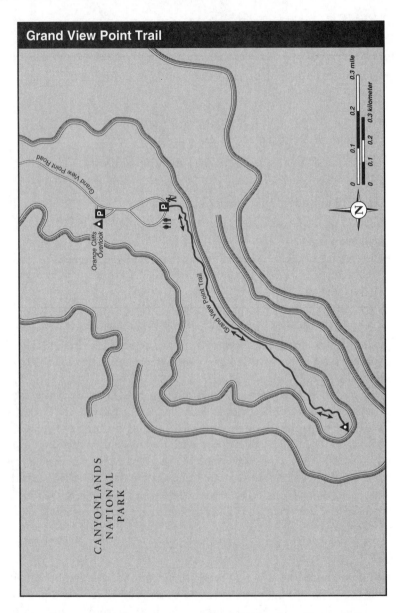

continually on your left. The route is clearly defined and beautifully manicured in stone. Junipers and piñons cling tenaciously to cliff walls. Almost the entire length of the path stays within about 20 feet of the unprotected cliff—not a comforting distance if you have small children who are inclined to run off at a moment's notice.

The trail remains flat and the hiking easy, making it a relaxing stroll. As you near the end of the point, cairns guide you to a promontory where the trail ends with nothing more than a precipitous drop-off, which is very different from what you might see in other national parks. The views are indeed grand, and no guardrails, fencing, or BEWARE OF CLIFF signs block the view. Enjoy it at a safe distance before returning the way you came.

TO THE TRAILHEAD
GPS Coordinates: N38º 18.643' W109º 51.397'
From the Island in the Sky Visitor Center, drive south for 12 miles along Grand View Point Road to the Grand View Point Overlook Parking Area.

JOHN WESLEY POWELL, EXPLORER OF THE AMERICAN WEST

John Wesley Powell's passion for the natural sciences and exploration was demonstrated early in his life as he rowed down the length of the Mississippi, Ohio, and Illinois Rivers while still in his early 20s. As a Union soldier in the Civil War, he was a cartographer and engineer before losing an arm at the Battle of Shiloh. Still, he continued to serve in many subsequent campaigns and attained the rank of major and lieutenant colonel.

After the war Powell had a professorship at Illinois State University, but his thirst for exploration led him to mount an expedition down the Green and Colorado Rivers, including the first passage through a chasm considered impassable by American Indians. Powell named that chasm the Grand Canyon.

Through Powell's extensive exploration of the American West and in his later position as director of the U.S. Geological Survey, he was instrumental in shaping the government's policy in the development of the region and approaches for managing critical issues related to settlement, water, grazing, mining, agriculture, forestry, and American Indian relations.

25 White Rim Overlook Trail

Trailhead Location: White Rim Overlook Parking Area

Trail Use: Walking, hiking

Distance & Configuration: 1.8-mile out-and-back

Elevation Range: 6,270' at trailhead to 6,100' at overlook

Facilities: Vault toilets and picnic tables at trailhead; no water

Highlights: A short, level walk to a scenic overview

DESCRIPTION

The White Rim Overlook sits on the opposite side of Island in the Sky from the Murphy Point Overlook, so while the far-ranging vistas are comparable—canyons, mesas, and cliffs—the views here are in the opposite direction. As a result, you have some beautiful La Sal scenes, as well as a glimpse into the gaping canyon of the Colorado River that you won't find on Murphy Point Trail. The distance from the rim overlook to the Colorado spans 2,000 vertical feet—about half of what you'll see in the Grand Canyon, but still quite impressive.

From the south rim of Island in the Sky, you can see what looks like an industrial site;—this is a potash mine that lies outside the confines of Canyonlands National Park near Moab. The other common view from the White Rim Overlook and many of the other overlooks is of the extensive network of winding dirt roads below the rim. Many of these backcountry roads had their origins as mining roads before the area became a national park. In addition to being a haven for hikers, all three districts of Canyonlands are immensely popular with mountain bikers and owners of four-wheel-drive vehicles. White Rim Road, which you'll see from this overlook, is especially popular, though less challenging than some of the other roads in the park.

Among the various overlooks in Island in the Sky, White Rim offers more solitude than most, so if your goal is to have an Edward Abbey *Desert Solitaire* experience, you've come to the right place.

ROUTE

Departing southbound from the trailhead picnic area, the trail descends slightly and, at 0.1 mile, comes to a signed junction where you'll take the

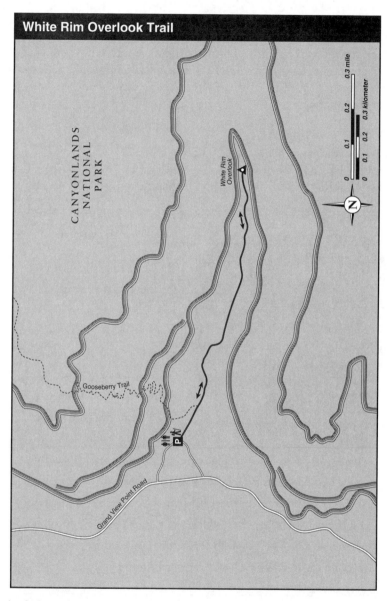

White Rim Overlook Trail

right fork in the direction of the White Rim. Already, views of the White Rim area begin to appear on the horizon, but the scenery only gets better as you approach the overlook.

The route combines an easy-to-follow trail with cairns, which makes route-finding a snap. Scattered Utah junipers adorn the plateau, along with fewer piñon pines than what you might find in other parts of the plateau. At 0.5 mile the dirt trail concedes to amply cairned slickrock and continues to a promontory distinguished by a small pinnacle and the overlook, at 0.9 mile. Before you return, you might feel that spirit of kinship with the settlers who first experienced these same views—largely unchanged—more than 100 years ago.

TO THE TRAILHEAD
GPS Coordinates: N38º 19.372' W109º 50.967'
From the Island in the Sky Visitor Center, drive 11.2 miles south on Grand View Point Road to the White Rim Overlook Parking Area, on your left.

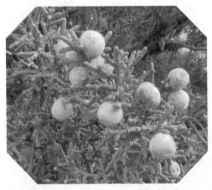

On a juniper tree, what appear to be berries are actually cones.

JUNIPER

The Utah juniper tree thrives on the mesa tops between 4,500 and 6,500 feet of elevation. Some of the region's trees are more than 100 years old. Because of the dry climate it inhabits, the Utah juniper will go to great lengths to survive. During dry periods, this tree, much like the bristlecone pine, will cut off water and fluids from some of its branches to increase its chance of survival. Its small, waxy leaves are another water-saving adaptation that enables it to survive in a climate with less than 9 inches of rain per year. Early settlers, as well as local residents today, sometimes called these trees cedars because the wood smells like cedar when cut or mulched.

26 Murphy Point Trail

Trailhead Location: Murphy Point Trailhead in the Island in the Sky district

Trail Use: Walking, hiking

Distance & Configuration: 3.6-mile out-and-back

Elevation Range: 6,260' at trailhead to 6,060' at rim

Facilities: None

Highlights: A moderate, level walk to the Murphy Point Overlook with views of the Green River

DESCRIPTION

This route to the rim used to be Murphy Point Road, suitable for passenger cars and not simply high-clearance or four-wheel-drive vehicles. The road led to a small parking area 0.2 mile from the overlook at the rim. In 1996, the National Park Service converted the road to a trail to preserve the more natural character of the Island in the Sky district.

Because the trail used to be a road, it still has a roadlike feel. It's a wide, straight, level beeline for the rim, with limited scenic appeal until you reach the final 0.2 mile. Still, this great overlook offers commanding views of Junction Butte to the southwest, White Rim country to the west of Island in the Sky, and the Green River below.

ROUTE

From the dirt parking area, the trail takes off across the sparse pasture of the mesa top, mixed with cacti, sage, blackbrush, Mormon tea, and other high desert species. At 0.5 mile you come to a Y in the trail, where you'll bear right in the signed direction of Murphy Point Overlook.

As you continue toward the rim, the vegetation diversifies only a bit to include piñons and junipers. Then, as the trail nears the point, just beyond where the old Murphy Point Road once terminated in a small parking area, it continues onto sparsely cairned Kayenta slickrock. What was once a well-defined roadbed is now a vague and barely identifiable trail. But you need not fear getting lost, because you're only 0.2 mile from the rim. If you continue in the same direction, the only place you can arrive is at the rim of Murphy Point.

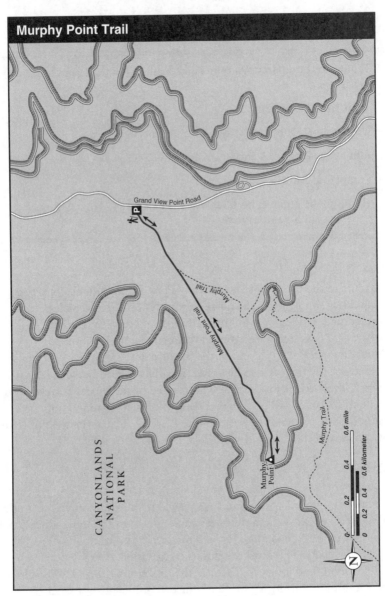

Murphy Point Trail

Once there, you can hike to two other overlooks, one to the east and another to the west. All offer great Canyonlands vistas, including the Abajo Mountains, the Henry Mountains, The Needles, and The Maze. For the best views of the Green River down below, the overlook to the west is your best choice. After admiring the scenery, make your way back to the trailhead.

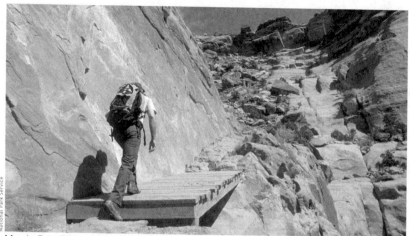

National Park Service

Murphy Point Trail

TO THE TRAILHEAD

GPS Coordinates: N38º 21.296' W109º 51.838'

From the Island in the Sky Visitor Center, drive 8.6 miles south on Grand View Point Road to the Murphy Point Parking Area, on your right.

WHAT IS THE GRAND STAIRCASE?

Extending from the Paunsaugunt Plateau in southern Utah (near Bryce Canyon) to the North Rim of the Grand Canyon, this amazing geologic feature is approximately 150 miles long and covers 6,000 vertical feet of elevation gain as it stretches north to south. In the 1870s, geologist Clarence Dutton described the area as a staircase extending out from the floor of the Grand Canyon. Each "step," or cliff, of the Grand Staircase extends up to 2,000 feet high. As you descend this stratigraphic staircase in your visit to the area, you travel back through time to ancient rock layers that are up to 600 million years old. Many of these layers are sandstone; some contain fossils of ancient life, while others may be composed of ancient lava rock.

27 Elephant Hill to Chesler Park

Trailhead Location: Elephant Hill Trailhead in the Needles district

Trail Use: Walking, hiking

Distance & Configuration: 5.8-mile out-and-back

Elevation Range: 5,124' at Elephant Hill Trailhead to 5,620' at Chesler Park Overlook

Facilities: None

Highlights: A hike with varied terrain and fascinating natural features; a superb introduction to the Needles District in a short hike

DESCRIPTION

This hike captures what many regard as the best of the Needle district's varied landscape. The formations you'll see make up only the outer edge of many more needlelike pinnacles and parallel canyons that extend to the Colorado River. Canyonlands' Needles were formed by a series of stress fractures in the rock surface caused by movement along a deep underlying layer of salt. Erosion by rainwater and snow along the fracture lines resulted in these rows of columnar rocks.

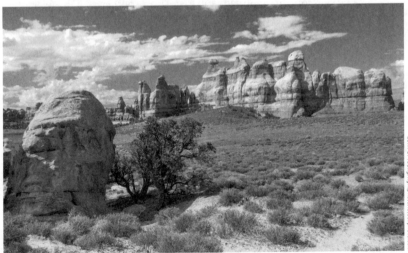

Colin D. Young/flightphoto/istockphoto.com

Chesler Park

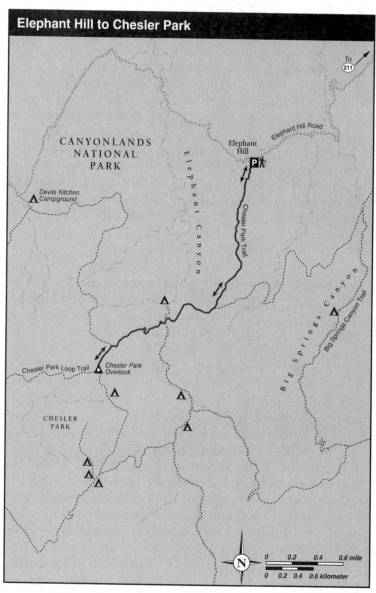

Elephant Hill to Chesler Park

CANYONLANDS
NATIONAL
PARK

Devils Kitchen
Campground

Elephant
Hill

Elephant Hill Road

To
211

Elephant Canyon

Chesler Park Trail

Big Springs Canyon

Big Springs Canyon Trail

Chesler Park Loop Trail

Chesler Park
Overlook

CHESLER
PARK

N

| 0 | 0.2 | 0.4 | 0.6 mile |
| 0 | 0.2 | 0.4 | 0.6 kilometer |

In this short hike you'll discover an area that's irresistibly appealing for backpackers looking for a longer stay, and you'll want to return for a two-, three-, or four-day adventure. Although the destination for this hike is Chesler Park, a wide-open expanse of grassland rimmed by the spires and slickrock formation of the Needles district, this route only goes as far as the rim of Chesler Park to an overview on the north side. The highlight and "wow" factor of this hike is the slickrock, the cracks, and the varied formations along the way, more than the view at the end. But this short jaunt will surely whet your appetite for more hiking in the Needles.

The route is primarily slickrock and provides a wonderful introduction to what makes the Needles district such a paradise for hikers and backpackers. This hike, along with most of the hiking in this section of Canyonlands, is replete with trail junctions, so for anything beyond the most basic park trails, you'll want to go equipped with a good hiking map of the area and the good sense to know how to use it. Water is also in short supply here, so you'll want to fill up before arriving at the trailhead and carry an ample supply with you. If you're properly equipped, and you have enough water and ample time, you could stretch this short hike into a 10- to 12-mile journey to include some exceptional other routes in the area.

ROUTE

The Elephant Hill Trailhead is a popular jumping-off point for both hikers and off-road vehicles. Hikers will be taking off on the trailhead at the southeast side of the parking area, while rough-terrain vehicles will be wrangling their way up the rock-strewn Elephant Hill Road. The hiking trail makes its first ascent on stone steps set between two house-size blocks of sandstone. Once you've gained your initial ascent from the trailhead, you arrive at a fanciful landscape of domes, towers, hoodoos, and balanced rocks sculpted in sandstone. You cross this section on a cairned route mixing slickrock, sand, and compacted dirt.

About 30 minutes from the trailhead, you'll come to the first of several junctions and a sign pointing to Chesler Park to the right, at 1.4 miles. Departing from the sign in the direction of Chesler Park, the trail climbs a narrow cleft between two immense mounds and eventually enters a crack between two sheer rock walls. Emerging from the crack, you'll continue, now on a descent into Elephant Canyon, where you bottom out in a wash. A sign near the wash identifies the location as Elephant Canyon and directs you to Chesler Park, at 0.8 mile ahead.

Exiting the wash in the direction of Chesler Park, you're surrounded by pinnacles on all sides, and you soon come to a sign directing you to Chesler Park, at 0.2 mile on your left. Arriving at the top of the hill, you have Chesler Park spread out in front of you; a sign on your left directs you to the viewpoint. Here your options are many, but if you have limited time in the Needles district and want to keep this as a short introductory hike, then your best option is to make the short ascent to the viewpoint, sit down, pull out a snack, and enjoy the view. Return to the trailhead the way you came, paying extra attention at each trail junction and saving other adventures and trails in the Needles for another day.

TO THE TRAILHEAD

GPS Coordinates: N38º 8.495' W109º 49.639'

From the Needles Visitor Center, continue west on Scenic Drive for 2.7 miles. Turn left at the junction signed to Elephant Hill. At 0.2 mile, turn right and continue another 0.2 mile. Veer to the right onto the dirt road, in the direction marked to Elephant Hill. After 2.7 miles on this well-graded dirt road, you reach the Elephant Hill Parking Area and Trailhead.

CONTROLLING THE INSECT POPULATION ONE GULP AT A TIME

Mosquitoes and other biting insects really are quite rare in the desert Southwest, and much of the credit goes to bats. A bat is capable of eating 30–100% of its body weight in a single evening. That's a lot of mosquitoes, scorpions, beetles, moths, crickets, and other pests. Along with their eyesight, bats use echolocation for navigation and to find their prey.

Canyonlands National Park is home to 16 native species of bats and is considered an excellent habitat for them. If you're near one of the water flows at dusk, you have an excellent chance of spotting one of these amazing creatures diving down to take a sip of water before it hunts for its evening meal.

---

28 Slickrock Trail

Trailhead Location: Slick Foot Trail Parking Area in the Needles district

Trail Use: Walking, hiking

Distance & Configuration: 2.4-mile balloon with short spurs to viewpoints

Elevation Range: 4,994' at roadside trailhead to 5,165' at the extension of loop

Facilities: None

Highlights: A cairn-marked loop trail over slickrock with some up close canyon views and distant views to the La Sal Mountains

DESCRIPTION

Slickrock is a defining feature of this region. Some of the most popular hiking trails, mountain biking routes, and campsites are set in slickrock. Most avid hikers in the Southwest relish slickrock trails for their undulating terrain, fascinating rock formations, and unobstructed views. Slickrock trails can also dish out some routefinding and navigational challenges. But for most hikers, reading the route and watching for a few well-placed cairns is part of the fun.

This short trail, almost entirely on rolling slickrock sandstone, offers the

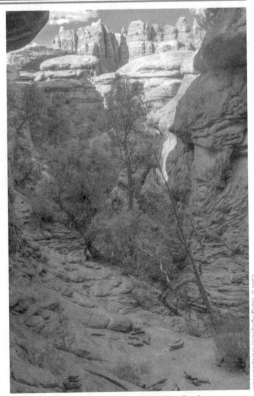

Elephant Canyon in Canyonlands' Needles district

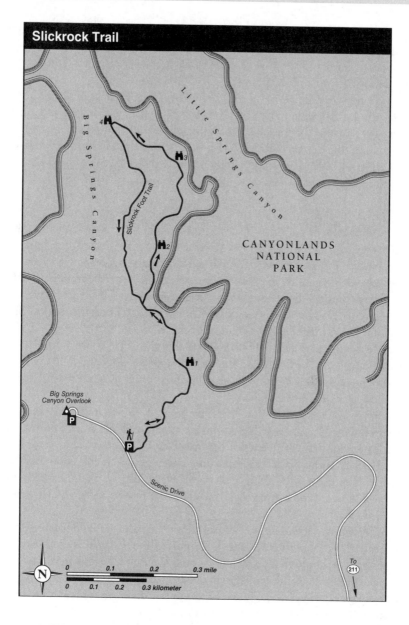

novice hiker an opportunity to discover the joys and challenges of slickrock hiking in a relatively easy-to-navigate setting. It's a great trek for younger hikers looking to build navigation skills and learning to follow cairns and subtle trail markings. In much the same way as those connect-the-dots puzzles you did as a child, you'll be hiking from cairn to cairn with three panoramic viewpoints along the way. At each viewpoint, signs let you know you're on the right track and provide valuable interpretive details about the area in which you're hiking.

Along the trail and at the viewpoints, you'll have views of Island in the Sky, the La Sal Mountains, the Needles, Big Springs Canyon, and Little Springs Canyon. Bighorn sheep may sometimes be spotted along the rock slopes or in the canyon bottoms. Because sightings are rare and the park likes to keep track of the bighorn population, you're asked to report any sheep you see to a park ranger.

ROUTE

From the roadside parking area, the trail dips from the road level and takes off to the north. It quickly arrives at slickrock outcrops dotted with junipers and piñons. An easy ascent takes you to the first viewpoint, with vistas of the La Sal Mountains to the northeast and the Abajo Mountains to the southeast. Both ranges are igneous formations that rose through layers of softer, more easily eroded sandstone. Eight miles to the east, you'll see Six-Shooter Peak, topped with its cluster of six spires.

Returning to the main trail, you'll follow the cairns to the north before arriving at a fork at 0.5 mile. Stay to the right to enter the loop counterclockwise; this allows you to follow the interpretive pamphlet available in the box near the trailhead.

Soon you'll see the sign for Viewpoint 2, which requires that you descend a bit, traverse a ledge, and then ascend a small knoll from which you'll be rewarded with views of Little Springs Canyon.

Return to the main trail, and then continue north and counterclockwise to Viewpoint 3. It affords views of Lower Little Springs Canyon, with its layers of gray and purple rock that color the mesas, cliffs, and slickrock knolls below.

Departing Viewpoint 3, the trail leads east along the longest spur of the trail; this part of the path is also the most difficult route-finding section. Arriving at Viewpoint 4, you'll enjoy grand views into Big Springs Canyon, 600 feet below. This is the most impressive of the four overlooks, with hanging gardens on the cliffs below and vistas of Grand View Point and Junction Butte rising high above Big Springs Canyon.

Departing Viewpoint 3, you'll head south and slightly to the west of the spur you took to get to Viewpoint 4. As you traverse cross-bedded layers of sandstone, pay close attention to the cairns and other evidences of trail use.

Continue in a southerly direction before completing the loop and retracing your final 0.5-mile leg back to the trailhead from which you started.

TO THE TRAILHEAD
GPS Coordinates: N38º 10.623' W109º 48.867'
From the Needles Visitor Center, take Scenic Drive west for 6.2 miles to the Slickrock Foot Trail Parking Area, on the right side of the road.

IT'S A HAWK! IT'S MY CELL PHONE!
OH, IT'S JUST A STELLER'S JAY.

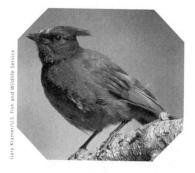

With personalities as colorful as their feathers, Steller's jays are abundant in Utah. These birds can be identified by their black crest and deep-blue feathers. Bird-watchers are often frustrated by these jays because they are excellent at mimicking other birds. Steller's jays frequently impersonate red-tailed hawks and other birds of prey to scare off birds from feeding areas. They've even been known to imitate people's cell-phone rings.

Gary Kramer/U.S. Fish and Wildlife Service

29 Horseshoe Canyon

Trailhead Location: Horseshoe Canyon Trailhead in the Horseshoe Canyon unit of the remote Maze district

Trail Use: Walking, hiking

Distance & Configuration: 6.8-mile out-and-back to the Great Gallery

Elevation Range: 5,341' at Horseshoe Canyon Trailhead to 4,800' at the Great Gallery

Facilities: Vault toilets at trailhead; no water

Highlights: Horseshoe Canyon is the Louvre of prehistoric rock art in the United States.

DESCRIPTION

Horseshoe Canyon is a popular and well-known destination among avid hikers in Utah, though it's rarely explored by out-of-state visitors. It's part of a detached unit of Canyonlands National Park, so it's not located near a visitor center, park entrance station, or any other town or public facility. In short, it's about as remote a location as you'll find in the contiguous United States. You really have to go out of your way to visit Horseshoe Canyon, so the hikers you encounter on the trail tend to be serious and sophisticated.

What they're usually after is the chance to stand in front of the Grand Gallery, a 200-foot-long panel featuring the finest example of prehistoric American Indian rock art in the United States. The panel portrays dozens of human and animal figures in red, brown, and white paint. The rock art is at least 2,000 years old, and possibly as old as 7,000 years; no one is really certain because this art is difficult to date. The work was created by archaic peoples who lived in the area before the arrival of the ancestral Pueblo culture (also called Anasazi), who occupied the area from roughly AD 100–1600, and before the Fremont culture, which flourished AD 700–1300. About 9 miles from Horseshoe Canyon, anthropologists have found clay figurines that are similar in style to the Great Gallery art and date to 4,700 BC.

The paintings were made from pigments comprised of finely ground minerals, mostly hematite, which were mixed with a liquid base such as animal fat or vegetable juice. In the thousands of years since the paintings were created, the base materials have disappeared, but the coloring still adheres to the rock with amazing clarity and definition.

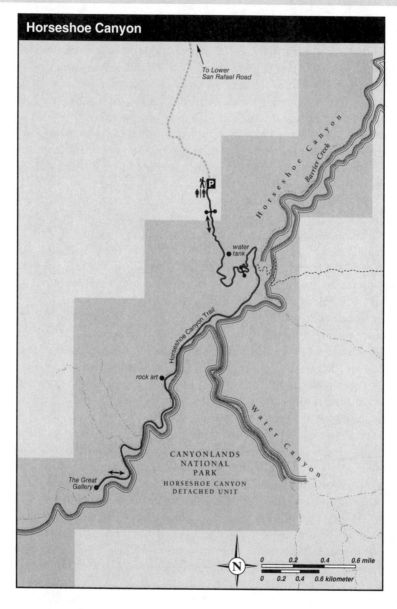

The humanlike figures in the Great Gallery, with their mummy forms, crowns, bulging eyes, and other inexplicable features, have mystified researchers. The dominant figure, known as the Holy Ghost—a 7-foot-tall painting with an ethereal appearance—is placed near the center of the Great Gallery. Is this a deity, a ruler, or a respected ancestor? Ponder such questions as you stand in the wash gazing at the Great Gallery.

ROUTE

From the parking area, make a quick descent into the canyon below on an old jeep road. The road was built and used by the Phillips Petroleum Company beginning in the 1920s. The rusted iron gate at 0.2 mile was later put up to keep vehicles from entering the canyon. At 0.5 mile from the trailhead, you'll come to an old tank and trough, the remains of a pumping system installed by sheep ranchers in the 1940s to bring water from the canyon to the pastures on the rim. The system never worked as planned and was abandoned shortly after it was installed. In this area it's also possible to see fossilized dinosaur tracks in the slickrock.

At 1.0 mile you'll come to a gate and wire fence with a sign communicating a stern reminder to not touch anything or deface the rock art. This gate features a viewpoint at a totally exposed and unprotected cliff, with dramatic views into the wash below. Descend below the gate along the crest of a sandy hill leading down into the wash—and consider that your ascent might be more grueling in a few hours when you're hot and tired.

At 1.3 miles from the trailhead, you arrive at the wash, where you will veer right and continue up the wash. It's so flat that you can barely tell whether you're ascending or descending, but by observing the vegetation in the wash, bent in the direction of the water flow during flash floods, it's easy to tell that you're walking uphill. During most of the year, you won't see any water flowing in the wash—just a few seeps and occasional small ponds in shaded spots. Within this deep canyon, you can enjoy the natural acoustics provided by the immense amphitheaters above you.

You'll continue up the wash with its constant turns, and you'll soon start thinking that the Great Gallery is surely just beyond the next one. But hiking in a sandy wash often forces a slower pace, and you don't always go as far as you think you have. At 0.8 mile up the wash, you come to a marked spur trail on the right that leads to a panel of rock art. It's not the Great Gallery, but rather a pleasant site in an alcove where the rock art has unfortunately suffered some damage, both natural and man-made.

At 3.4 miles from the trailhead, and after walking for 2.1 miles in the wash, you arrive at the Great Gallery, on your right. On weekends and during some of the busier times of the year, an interpretive ranger is at the site to discuss the history and culture of the peoples who created the art. But whether or not a ranger is present, you'll want to allow ample time for this impressive panel to stir your imagination and arouse your feelings for the ancient Indians who dwelled in this desert canyon.

TO THE TRAILHEAD

GPS Coordinates: N 38º 28.417' W 110º 12.023'

Horseshoe Canyon is in the Maze district, to the east of both the Green River and the Colorado River, the most remote and least-visited section of Canyonlands National Park. Rather than accessing this area from Moab, you'll need to be on UT 24, coming from either Hanksville to the south or from I-70 and the town of Green River to the north.

Coming from Green River, Utah, take I-70 west for 15 miles to Exit 147 (Utah 24/Hanksville). Turn left at the end of the off-ramp and go south on UT 24. Proceed south on UT 24, passing the entrance to Goblin Valley State Park on the right and continuing another 0.5 mile to turn left on a dirt road signed for the Hans Flat Ranger Station. From the turnoff to the first junction is 24 miles on a graded dirt road. At this fork, you'll see a sign for a road to the right that goes to Hans Flat—instead, take the fork to the left, which goes to Horseshoe Canyon. Continue another 5.5 miles from the junction to a road on the right, signed for Horseshoe Canyon. The Horseshoe Canyon Trailhead is in a large parking area at the end of this road, 1.5 miles from the turn.

ANCIENT MESSAGES

If you look closely at many of the cliff faces, you may see pictures of people, animals, and other designs on the walls. These are petroglyphs and pictographs created by the area's early inhabitants, such as the Fremont, Anasazi, and other Paleo Indians. Many petroglyphs tell stories, while others provided directions or instructions. We have not yet deciphered some petroglyphs; perhaps they were giving us a message. If you do see this marvelous rock art, please take nothing but pictures, and leave the art undisturbed for future visitors to discover and enjoy.

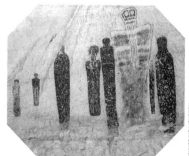

The famous Holy Ghost Panel

National Park Service

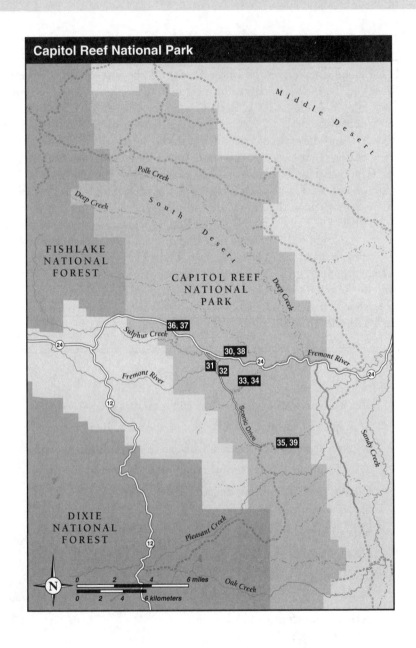

Capitol Reef National Park

CAPITOL REEF NATIONAL PARK

Park Overview

Established in 1971 to preserve the desert landscape around the Waterpocket Fold, a 100-mile-long wrinkle in the earth's crust, Capitol Reef National Park is a hidden gem. Ask most locals to name the five national parks in Utah, and Capitol Reef is usually the last one mentioned, if not forgotten completely. It's an unheralded treasure—a true hiker's park, not just a series of shuttle stops and overviews.

To experience and appreciate its magnificent scenery, get out of the car and do some walking or, better yet, backpacking in the park's expansive backcountry. You'll discover a colorful array of arches, natural bridges, domes, canyons, and cliffs, all weathered and eroded by the forces of wind, water, time, and the harsh extremes of the desert climate. You'll be hooked, and you'll want to come back for more.

Capitol Reef also celebrates the human history of a region centered on the agricultural abundance made possible by the Fremont River, which cuts through the Waterpocket Fold before emptying into the Colorado River. The indigenous Fremont people, who lived in the region for nearly 600 years, left behind pictographs, petroglyphs, and granaries. More recently, Mormon pioneers in the 1880s founded the community of Fruita and devised an irrigation system to water thousands of fruit trees. Today the visitor center, the campground, and many of the park's best hikes are clustered around the Fruita Rural Historic District, where a restored one-room school, farmhouse, and barn re-create life in a small agricultural community.

JUST ONE DAY?

By staying in the nearby town of Torrey, just west of the park, you can get an early start on the day at Capitol Reef. Don't miss Hickman Bridge, the park's most popular hike, before visiting Fruita and the Gifford farmhouse. Then have lunch in the Fruita picnic area. For an afternoon hike, it's a toss-up between Cassidy Arch and the longer Sulphur Creek route—though if you choose Sulphur Creek, you'll want to plan ahead and arrange a shuttle to the trailhead.

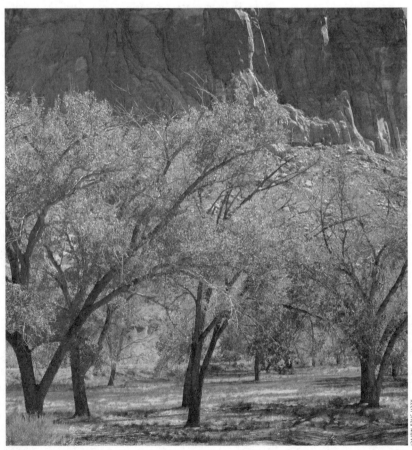

Cottonwood trees are abundant in riparian regions of the Southwest. See the sidebar on page 134.

30 Hickman Bridge

Trailhead Location: Parking area on the north side of UT 24 and the Fremont River, just 2.0 miles east of Capitol Reef Visitor Center

Trail Use: Walking, hiking

Distance & Configuration: 2.2-mile balloon

Elevation Range: 5,357' at trailhead to 5,707' near Hickman Bridge

Facilities: Vault toilets at trailhead; no water

Highlights: A slickrock-and-sand trail leads through a beautiful natural bridge.

DESCRIPTION

The Hickman Bridge Trail is the most popular hike in the park, but don't let that keep you from enjoying its wonders. In off-the-beaten-path Capitol Reef, it's possible that you could be alone much of the way.

In fact, Hickman Natural Bridge is used to being lonely. It remained hidden to early settlers and wasn't discovered until 1940—surprisingly late,

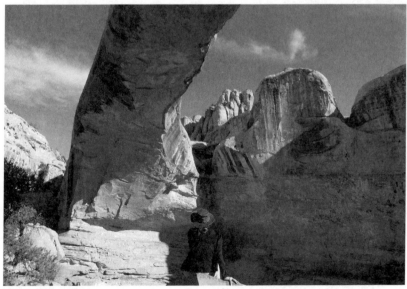

Hickman Natural Bridge

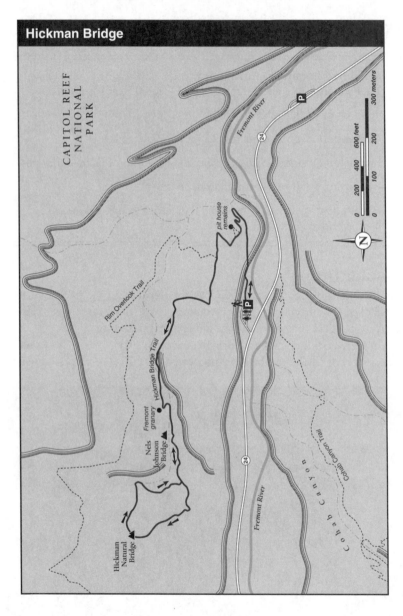

Hickman Bridge

considering that the surrounding area was a pocket of Fremont culture activity and pioneer farming. Once discovered, the bridge was named in honor of Joe Hickman, a Torrey educator who spent much of his life working to get Capitol Reef designated as a national monument.

The trail offers plenty of visual interest and variety. In addition to the namesake bridge, you'll see the stone foundation of a Fremont pit house and the remains of a cliffside granary. The trail includes stretches of cottonwood-shaded riverside, steeply ascending steps, slickrock, sand, a narrows, and the 133-foot-long Hickman Natural Bridge—all of which should keep any child and most adults fully entertained and engaged. The trail is largely exposed to full sun in the summer, so plan ahead by taking along ample water and protection from the sun.

ROUTE

Before setting out on the trail, pick up one of the interpretive flyers from a metal box at the east side of the trailhead parking area. The flyer provides information about the natural and cultural history of the hike and corresponds with the 17 numbered markers along the trail.

From the trailhead parking area, walk east toward the rushing flow of the river and through well-watered cottonwoods. With the Fremont River to your right and a rugged Kayenta Formation red cliff on your left, you pass through riparian underbrush of willows and tamarisks.

After a few minutes, the cover of shade comes to an end as the trail cuts to the left and makes a hairpin turn to begin its steep ascent on a well-designed and maintained track, with steps crafted from quarried blocks of sandstone. The steps lead to dry benchland terrain that is characteristic of much of the hiking within Capitol Reef. Ascending these steps, you'll have fine views of Capitol Dome and the river valley below.

At trail marker 4, the trail forks right on a spur to the northeast. At about 50 feet you'll discover a ring of black boulders, which is the remains of a pit house, the typical home built by the Fremont people. Be sure to stay on the trail and avoid walking on or disturbing any of the material in this archeological site. Continuing on the main trail beyond the pit house foundation, you'll come to a junction with the Rim Overlook–Navajo Knobs Trail on your right. Continue straight in the marked direction of Hickman Natural Bridge.

Soon the trail descends into a sandy wash as the canyon walls rise above. As you pass through a stretch of sand, cast your gaze to the right to spot a cliffside alcove cradling the remains of a Fremont granary, perhaps 700 years old or more. A diverse variety of desert plants—including yucca, Utah serviceberry, prickly pear cactus, and 20 different species of wildflowers in season—dot the hillside and wash.

Another minute past the granary and you'll see Nels Johnson Bridge, named for an early Fruita homesteader, spanning the wash bottom. Passing the Johnson Bridge, the trail splits at 0.8 mile (5,600 feet elevation) to form a loop that approaches Hickman Natural Bridge. Stay to the left for now and you'll rejoin the trail at this point after completing the loop.

Soon Hickman Natural Bridge comes into full view. It's a magnificent span of tan Kayenta Sandstone, one of the largest in Capitol Reef National Park, measuring 125 feet in height and with a span of 133 feet. Walk under the bridge and do your best to follow the faint trail along the slickrock ledges beyond the bridge. You'll soon find yourself on a more distinguishable trail that returns you to the loop junction and back to the trailhead.

TO THE TRAILHEAD
GPS Coordinates: N38º 17.325' W111º 13.656'
From the Capitol Reef Visitor Center, continue east on UT 24 for 2.0 miles. The trailhead parking area is on the north side of the road.

COTTONWOODS: THEIR FEET IN THE WATER

Throughout the Southwest, the most abundant shade tree is the cottonwood (*Populus*). And because it grows naturally only in wet soils, typically along streams and rivers, its presence was a sign to parched desert travelers that water was nearby. Many of the mature cottonwoods along the Fremont River and in Fruita have trunks measuring 2–5 feet in diameter. In the heat of summer, these trees can consume and transpire up to 400 gallons of water per day.

Their root systems protect against riverbank erosion, their canopy provides a shaded and moister environment for other plants and animals, and their strong branches offer a nesting habitat for great blue herons. But as a result of livestock grazing, clear-cutting, and waterway diversion, more than 90% of the Southwest's once-abundant cottonwood forests are now gone.

31 Fremont River Trail

Trailhead Location: Near the Fruita picnic area or on Loop B of the Fruita Campground

Trail Use: Walking, hiking; also wheelchair-accessible, pets, cycling (for the first 0.6 mile)

Distance & Configuration: 2.7-mile out-and-back from the Fruita picnic area or 2.1-mile out-and-back from the Fruita Campground

Elevation Range: 5,425' at the Fremont River near the Gifford Homestead to 5,905' at the ridgetop

Facilities: Restrooms and water in the Gifford Homestead and the Fruita Campground

Highlights: A representative slice of the park—the river, orchards, campground, canyon, cliffs, and a mesa with panoramic views

DESCRIPTION

Are you staying in Fruita Campground and looking for an invigorating early morning walk? Are you searching for a hike that will give you some energizing elevation gain, the restorative sound of rushing water, and inspirational views? The Fremont River Trail is accessible from the Fruita picnic area, the Gifford Homestead, and the Fruita Campground and may be the wake-up call for which you're looking, or it may be the perfect introductory hike if you're staying in the park a couple days or more. If you're an early-morning birder or photographer, or if you want to walk a less-traveled path that is still in the heart of the park, just a few minutes by car from the visitor center, then this is your hike.

The first 0.5 mile of the hike is the park's only wheelchair-accessible trail, and it's also a relaxing riverside stroll, where you'll have the Fremont River continually by your side. The Fremont River is a ribbon of greenery and life that bisects the arid and rocky topography of Capitol Reef. On this trail you'll pass through productive orchards and see some of the rusted skeletons of vintage farm machinery. Then you ascend a rocky cliff overlooking a canyon before topping out on a quiet mesa where the vistas extend farther to the east.

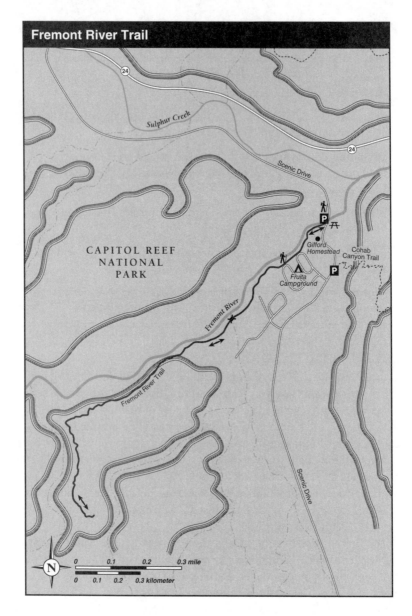

Fremont River Trail

Sulphur Creek

24

Scenic Drive

24

CAPITOL REEF
NATIONAL
PARK

Gifford
Homestead

Cohab
Canyon Trail

Fruita
Campground

Fremont River

Fremont River Trail

Scenic Drive

0   0.1   0.2   0.3 mile

0   0.1   0.2   0.3 kilometer

N

ROUTE

The Fremont River Trail offers two convenient starting points: the Fruita
picnic area and the amphitheater parking area in the Fruita Campground.
If you've just arrived in the park and are leaving the visitor center, then the

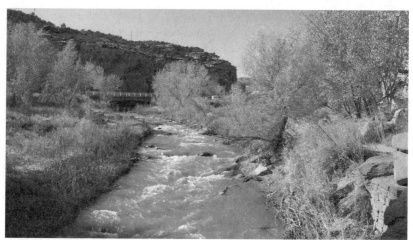

The Fremont River—bringing life to the desert

picnic area is the logical starting point. But if you're staying in the Fruita Campground, you can just as easily walk from your campsite toward the river and quickly connect with the trail.

Starting from the picnic area and crossing Campground Drive at the crosswalk, you'll see a sign marking the trailhead. You're on the south bank of the gurgling Fremont River. With the river on your right and the Gifford Homestead about 100 yards in front of you, start your way down this wide, graded path. You'll soon pass behind the Gifford Homestead, and within a minute or so you'll have the amphitheater, pear and apple orchards, and a horse pasture on your left. At 0.3 mile from the trailhead. you come to a box where you can purchase a Fremont River Trail interpretive pamphlet. This is also the point where you connect with the trail if you're starting in the campground.

With peach and apricot orchards on your left and tall reed grasses on your right, continue your way upstream. Be on the lookout for wildlife, as mule deer are common in the meadows of Fruita and beaver, skunks, and marmots find lush habitat in the riverside grasses and thickets. In the early-morning hours, this area is also ideal for birding. Soon the path crosses a sturdy wooden bridge spanning an irrigation ditch at 0.4 mile from the trailhead.

At 0.6 mile, the wheelchair-accessible portion of the trail comes to an end. The trail narrows and a sign advises NO BIKES OR DOGS BEYOND THIS POINT. The path begins a serious ascent, hugging the wall of the mesa to the right as it moves upward through the red ledges of a Moenkopi cliff. At 1.0 mile. you come to a fine overlook on a promontory with views up the Fremont River and into a tributary canyon on the south.

As the trail curves to the south, the tributary canyon lies to your right. Switchbacks take you through yellowish layers of Sinbad Limestone and onto the ridge, where the trail concludes at a ridgetop overview at 1.3 miles.

The views of the campground and the Fruita orchards below are familiar, but the panoramic scenes stretching north to south will introduce you to some of the park's showpieces. The rounded Navajo Knobs lie north, the entrance to Cohab Canyon is in front of you, and the unmistakable Ferns Nipple can be seen to the south. The general horizon to the east is a particularly rugged section of the 100-mile-long Waterpocket Fold, Capitol Reef's defining geologic backbone.

Once you've had ample time to take in the vista and breathe the desert air, retrace your route to the campground or Fruita.

TO THE TRAILHEAD

GPS Coordinates: N38º 17.069' W111º 14.803'
From the Capitol Reef Visitor Center, go 1.0 mile south on Campground Road to the picnic parking area, on your left. The trail begins across the street, on the south side of the Fremont River.

FREMONT RIVER

The Fremont River is the only water flow to cut through the 100-mile-long Waterpocket Fold. Named for explorer John C. Fremont, it has a source high on the Wasatch Plateau near Fish Lake. As it descends toward Capitol Reef, it provides irrigation water for the farming communities of Loa, Bicknell, and Torrey, and it was the only water source for Fruita. After leaving Capitol Reef, the Fremont River joins with the Muddy River near Hanksville to form the Dirty Devil, which flows into the Colorado River.

---

32 Cohab Canyon

Trailhead Location: Cohab Canyon Trailhead on Scenic Drive

Trail Use: Walking, hiking

Distance & Configuration: 3.4-mile out-and-back or 1.7-mile point-to-point; additional 1.1-mile spur trail to both overlooks

Elevation Range: 5,340' at UT 24 trailhead to 5,760' at ridgetop overview above Fruita

Facilities: Restrooms and water nearby at Fruita Campground and Capitol Reef Visitor Center

Highlights: A scenic canyon in the heart of the park that connects with many other trails

DESCRIPTION

Capitol Reef is full of great nooks and crannies. The park's centerpiece, the Waterpocket Fold, is nothing more than a crinkle in the earth's crust that results in hundreds of natural-made hiding places in the form of slot canyons, arches, natural bridges, and fins. Before Butch Cassidy made his hideout here, Mormon polygamists, known as cohabitants ("cohabs" for short), found refuge in some of these canyons in the 1880s when polygamists were pursued as felons by US marshals. Cohab Canyon would have been a perfect shelter given its proximity to Fruita, its barely noticeable entrance, and its shady, hospitable setting.

Cohab Canyon is a popular stand-alone hike in Capitol Reef, or it can be added to many other trails within the park. With its central location, Cohab Canyon connects with Cassidy Arch, the Frying Pan Trail, and Grand Wash and can be used to link multiple short trails. But it's also a great hike in its own right. It's best done as a one-way hike, either starting in Fruita and following the canyon in its northeasterly descent to the Fremont River as described here, or, conversely, starting at the UT 24 trailhead and ascending the canyon in a southwesterly direction.

ROUTE

From the large stone sign marking the Fruita trailhead, you gain the hike's full elevation in the first 0.3 mile on 22 strenuous switchbacks through the clay mounds of the Chinle Formation. The steady ascent takes you to

Cohab Canyon

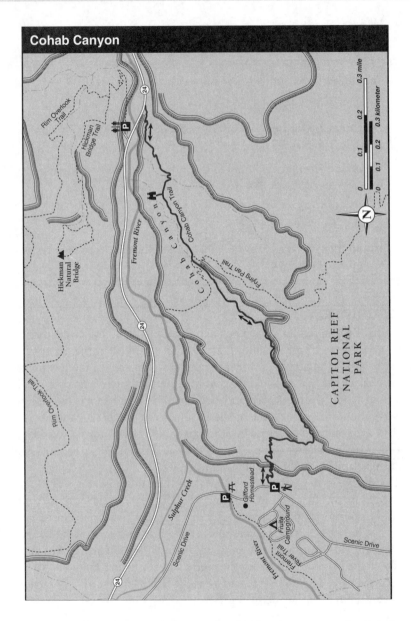

a ridgetop, the crest of the Waterpocket Fold, where at nearly 400 feet above Fruita, you have a great view into the campground. You're standing at the base of Wingate Sandstone cliffs, which you skirt on the west side before dropping into the main channel of Cohab Canyon.

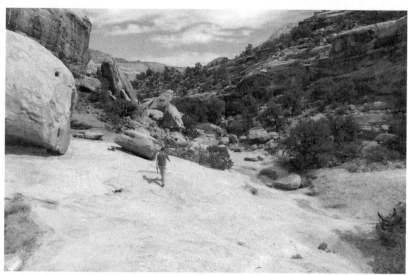

Cohab Canyon

Once you're in the canyon, the vegetation becomes more abundant and includes piñon, box elder, and single-leaf ash trees. Although bighorn sheep sightings are not commonplace in Capitol Reef, you have as good a chance of seeing them here in Cohab Canyon as any place in the park. Side slot canyons invite exploration, including one at 0.1 mile on the south (right) after entering the canyon. The trail stays in the wash, which is easy to follow. Then, at 0.8 mile from the trailhead, the trail moves from the wash onto a higher section of slickrock and into the lower half of the canyon.

At 1.0 mile a spur trail, signed FRUITA OVERLOOK, takes off to the left and requires climbing out of the canyon. The spur soon arrives at a fork, with the path on the left going to a south overlook and the path on the right leading to a north overlook. Visiting both overlooks, which is recommended, adds 1.1 miles to the hike, but it's a rewarding extension.

Returning to the canyon and crossing the wash, you'll soon arrive at the junction of the Frying Pan Trail. Stay straight. From here on, the trail stays above the wash. Nearing the mouth of the canyon, you'll have views of Capitol Dome, the cupola-shaped formation that gives Capitol Reef its name. On the right you'll also see Pectols Pyramid, a beautiful 6,970-foot peak set on the south side of UT 24.

Cohab Canyon empties into the Fremont River near the Hickman Bridge Trailhead on UT 24. Here you'll find restrooms, but no water other than that flowing in the Fremont. If you've left a shuttle vehicle at the

Hickman Bridge Trailhead, then you've arrived at your destination. Otherwise, retrace your steps back up Cohab Canyon, paying particular attention to the trail junctions and markings—it's especially easy to get off-trail and mistakenly wind up on the Frying Pan Trail on your return.

TO THE TRAILHEAD

GPS Coordinates: *Cohab Canyon Trailhead:* N38º 16.950' W111º 14.778'
UT 24 Trailhead: N38º 17.000' W111º 14.174'
From the Capitol Reef Visitor Center, drive south on Scenic Drive for 1.0 mile to the Cohab Canyon Trailhead, on the left side of the road opposite the Fruita Campground. Parking is available at the Gifford Homestead and in the picnic parking area just before the Gifford house. If you plan to do this as a one-way hike, arrange for a shuttle at the UT 24 trailhead. To get there from the Capitol Reef Visitor Center, continue east on UT 24 for 2.0 miles. The Hickman Bridge Parking Area is on the north side of the road, and the UT 24 trailhead is just a couple hundred feet farther on the south side of the road.

DESERT VARNISH

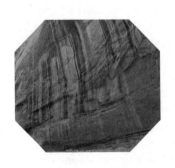 What sometimes looks like chocolate or butterscotch syrup dripping down from the rock is desert varnish, which is caused by precipitation of clay minerals containing oxides of iron and manganese as rainfall and groundwater evaporate from the rock face. Varnish is very thin and only forms in protected areas of rock, especially sandstone, where it is not eroded away by wind and water. Many American Indians created petroglyphs by chipping away the desert varnish to expose the lighter rock beneath.

33 Cassidy Arch

Trailhead Location: Grand Wash Trailhead

Trail Use: Walking, hiking

Distance & Configuration: 3.3-mile out-and-back

Elevation Range: 5,435' at Grand Wash Trailhead to 6,000' at Cassidy Arch overlook

Facilities: Vault toilet at trailhead

Highlights: A rollicking trail leading to a spectacular arch that can be walked upon

DESCRIPTION

For an avid hiker, Capitol Reef is one of the most appealing national parks in America, and Cassidy Arch is a showstopper in Capitol Reef. The trail offers the variety, the adventure, and the kind of culminating destination that every great hike should have. And at just 3.3 miles round-trip, it's a walk with broad appeal—experienced trekkers, families, and first-time hikers alike will find something to get excited about.

It's a front-country trail with a backcountry attitude. Named after outlaw Butch Cassidy, who reportedly had a hideout here, the trail is custom-made for a bank robber trying to evade the long arm of the law. You'll start with your boots in the sand and quickly make a surprise breakout onto cliffside switchbacks. You'll contour your way through intriguing and unnamed side canyons. A clever fork in the trail, marked only by a small cairn, guarantees that no footprints will be seen on the barren rock. You gaze down on the wash and road below from a vantage point shared with bighorn sheep and the elusive mountain lion. Finally, nearing the arch, the trail disappears and becomes just a rolling route over barren slickrock, and then instantly our arch appears in full view and you're standing above it. Get ready for some surprises.

ROUTE

With no water at the trailhead, no reliable water sources along the trail, and virtually no shade, you'll want to fill your bottles to the brim at the visitor center or in Fruita before heading down Scenic Drive. As you turn

Cassidy Arch

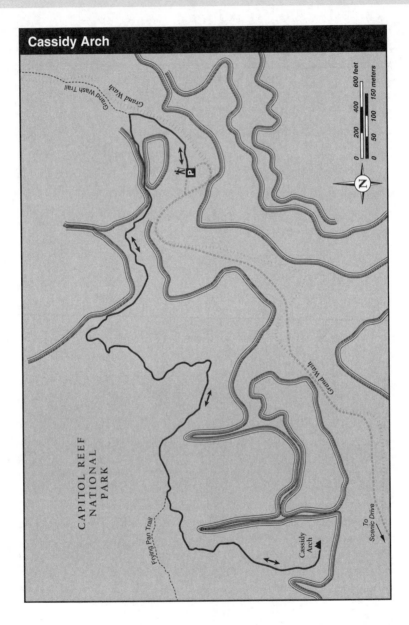

off Scenic Drive onto the dirt Grand Wash Road, look to the canyon walls on the north and notice the now-sealed uranium mine that's more than 100 years old. An interpretive sign on the north side of the dirt road recaps the barely profitable mining operations in the area.

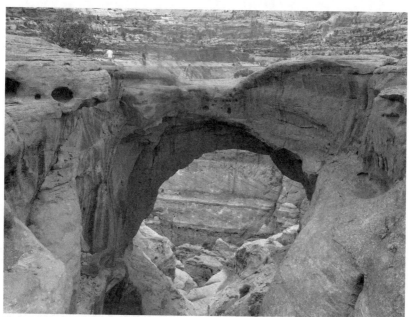

Cassidy Arch

From the small parking area at the end of Grand Wash Road, a short trail quickly connects you with the sandy, gravelly base of the wash. As you make your way down the wash, note the pocked canyon walls with cavities carved by rushing water—convincing evidence of the way water sculpts these desert canyons, and an indication of why the sign at the mouth of the canyon warns you not to enter when thunderstorms are predicted.

After 0.2 mile in the wash, you'll see a cairn-marked spur to the left and soon a sign reading CASSIDY ARCH TRAIL 1.5 MILES, ELEV. HERE 5,400, AT ARCH 6,350 (actually, though, the arch elevation is just under 6,000 feet). Follow this route as it quickly ascends the face of the canyon wall. It's a steep rise through Kayenta Formation ledges, where you'll find yourself winding around jumbled boulders and some tight switchbacks to gain a lot of elevation quickly. Soon the climb moderates a bit, and at 0.4 mile from the trailhead you'll have some satisfying views down into the wash.

You're likely to see bighorn sheep droppings on the trail, and early-morning hikers might even glimpse one of these canyon dwellers at close range. At about 1.0 mile from the trailhead, you'll have your first peek at Cassidy Arch in the distance to the left. You'll also have a fine view of Ferns Nipple, a cone of Navajo Sandstone to the south.

At 1.3 miles from the trailhead, you'll come to a fork in the trail with a sign directing you to Cassidy Arch on the left at 0.5 mile. From here on, the route rolls across slickrock, and the trail is evident only in occasional sandy pockets. Across this open expanse of slickrock is the occasional piñon and roundleaf buffaloberry.

Nearing the end of the trail, stay left of the rounded white outcrops. If this is your first visit, you may start to wonder where the arch is—then suddenly, it appears on your left. It's a delight and often a bit surprising, because most arches are viewed from below. But you'll be seeing Cassidy Arch from above. This rare vantage point allows you to safely cross over the top of the arch and take in some inspiring scenery. Before you return the way you came, venture over to the ledge about 100 feet to the south for some heart-pounding views straight down the canyon wall to the wash below.

TO THE TRAILHEAD

GPS Coordinates: N38º 15.826' W111º 12.940'
From the Capitol Reef Visitor Center, go south on Scenic Drive for 3.5 miles to the graded dirt road signed for Grand Wash. Turn left and continue east on Grand Wash Road for 1.3 miles to the trailhead parking area.

BUTCH CASSIDY SLEPT HERE

Robert Leroy Parker was born in Beaver, Utah, in 1866, the oldest of 13 children. In his early teens he worked for Mike Cassidy, a cattle rustler and horse thief, and later he took the name Butch Cassidy in honor of his friend and mentor. Butch Cassidy was known as one of the most notorious robbers in the American West. During the late 1800s, he robbed trains and banks and was involved in several shootouts. He was also the leader of the Wild Bunch Gang with his partner in crime, Harry Alonzo Longabaugh, better known as the Sundance Kid. The area now known as Capitol Reef National Park was one of Cassidy's hideouts while he was on the run. Cassidy was reportedly killed in a shootout in Bolivia in 1908.

34 Grand Wash

Trailhead Location: Grand Wash Trailhead east of Scenic Drive

Trail Use: Walking, hiking

Distance & Configuration: 4.8-mile out-and-back, 2.4-mile point-to-point, or 1.5-mile out-and-back from UT 24 trailhead to The Narrows and back

Elevation Range: 5,435' at Grand Wash Trailhead to 5,230' at the Fremont River

Facilities: Vault toilet at trailhead

Highlights: Sheer canyon walls, weathered and varnished, rise above the wash route.

DESCRIPTION

Grand Wash is one of only six drainages that slice through the Waterpocket Fold, and similar to Capitol Gorge, a walk down Grand Wash is a fairly leisurely jaunt, with little in the way of elevation gain along the floor of a desert canyon. The scenic appeal is found in the vertical canyon walls that tower above you on both sides. These Navajo Sandstone cliffs, weathered,

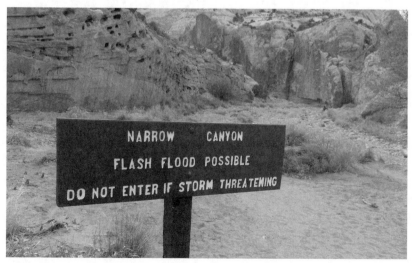

Take precautions when hiking in desert canyons.

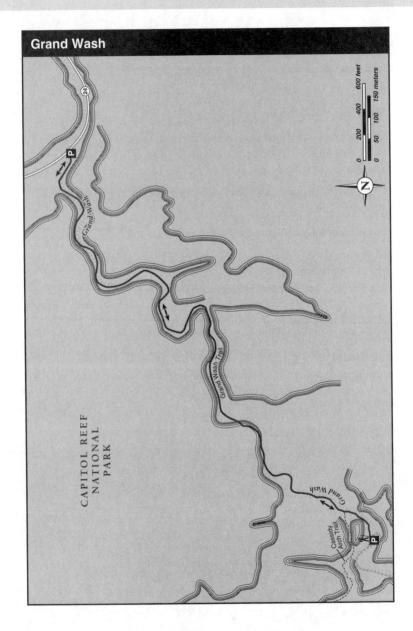

decorated with desert varnish, and pocked with solution cavities, rise 600–800 feet above the floor of the wash. The Narrows of Grand Wash constrict to a width of just 16 feet at one point and stretch for nearly 0.5 mile.

Grand Wash was created by water flowing through this fissure in the Waterpocket Fold, and the scouring of the canyon walls is clearly evident and quite impressive. Even though Grand Wash is subject to occasional flash flooding, the trail surface is hard-packed dirt rather than gravelly sand, so it makes for easier and more enjoyable walking than you'll find in some of the other nearby washes.

This hike can be tackled in several ways: as a round-trip from either the Grand Wash Trailhead or the UT 24 trailhead, as a one-way hike from either end, or as an out-and-back just as far as The Narrows from either trailhead. The Narrows are slightly closer to the UT 24 trailhead, so if you're after the shortest and fastest way to access The Narrows, park your vehicle at the marked UT 24 trailhead and make a quick out-and-back to The Narrows—though the vast majority of hikers start this route at the Grand Wash Trailhead.

ROUTE

From the elevated Grand Wash parking area, the trail stays above the wash for the first 0.1 mile and then drops into the wash, where you'll stay for the remainder of the hike. After 0.3 mile from the trailhead, a cairn-marked spur to the left directs you to Cassidy Arch and the Frying Pan Trail, but you'll stay in the wash and continue straight ahead.

At this point you're in the Kayenta Formation, with numerous alcoves and ledges dotted with piñons and junipers. After passing a rocky section about 1.0 mile from the trailhead, the route enters Navajo Sandstone, and the tightest section of The Narrows begins as the walls are separated by a spread of only 16 feet. The Narrows also features some flowing curves and continues for nearly 0.5 mile before the canyon widens again. As you exit The Narrows, the variety and abundance of vegetation, which includes Apache plume and serviceberry, increases.

The canyon continues to widen, and at 2.4 miles from the trailhead you'll arrive at UT 24, where a sign marks this alternate entrance to the wash. The Fremont River runs alongside the highway on the north. Here you can make your turnaround for the return to the Grand Wash Trailhead, or you can meet your planned shuttle pickup in one of the roadside parking places.

TO THE TRAILHEAD

GPS Coordinates: *Grand Wash Trailhead:* N38º 15.826' W111º 12.940'
UT 24 Trailhead: N38º 16.700' W111º 11.554'
From the Capitol Reef Visitor Center, go south on Scenic Drive for 3.5 miles to the graded dirt road signed to Grand Wash. Turn left and continue east on Grand Wash Road for 1.3 miles to the trailhead parking area. If you're starting at the UT 24 trailhead, take UT 24 east from the visitor center for 4.5 miles to the signed trailhead, on the right.

URANIUM MINING IN CAPITOL REEF

Long before the atomic bomb and the uranium boom of the 1950s, a claim was filed in 1904 on a site just north of Grand Wash Road. The two mine openings (now covered by metal doors) are visible from the dirt road about 0.1 mile east of Scenic Drive. Although uranium ore had limited value at that time, radium was one of the most precious minerals on Earth, worth about $80,000 per gram. Despite traces of radium that occurred as impurities in the uranium ore, the claim's production was small.

During the 1920s, uranium ore from this mine was ground up and mixed with drinking water or placed in packets over arthritic joints to cure rheumatism and other ailments—an early treatment that was likely more harmful than the disease it was intended to cure.

35 Golden Throne Trail

Trailhead Location: Capitol Gorge Trailhead

Trail Use: Walking, hiking

Distance & Configuration: 4.0-mile out-and-back

Elevation Range: 5,449' at Capitol Gorge Trailhead to 6,140' at TRAIL'S END sign

Facilities: Vault toilet and covered picnic tables at trailhead; no water

Highlights: Remote and scenic side canyon with dramatic views of some of Capitol Reef's signature formations

DESCRIPTION

Among Capitol Reef's front-country trails, the Golden Throne Trail is a less-frequented route that takes you from the floor of the canyon to scenic panoramas along the top of the Waterpocket Fold. In 2.0 miles, you'll gain 700 feet of elevation as you mount rugged ledges and traverse above cliffs.

Upon reaching the crest of the Waterpocket Fold, you'll be rewarded by views that stretch to the Aquarius Plateau and the Henry Mountains. Although the trail never really ascends the Golden Throne, it does offer some great vistas of this majestic monolith at close range. The Golden Throne is one of the most prominent domes in the park, rising 600 feet above the surrounding plateau.

With the elevation gain on this hike comes a wider variety of vegetation than you might find on other hikes in the park. Piñons and junipers are plentiful, as are Mormon tea and roundleaf buffaloberry.

When you've completed the hike and are driving back to the visitor center along Scenic Drive, stop at the Golden Throne viewpoint and take in the more distant view of this impressive slickrock dome. Pat yourself on the back for having made the ascent to its base.

ROUTE

The Capitol Gorge Road that leads to the trailhead is a well-maintained, 2.0-mile-long dirt road. Like many of the graded roads in the park, it can be hazardous and may be closed when thunderstorms threaten. Once at

Golden Throne Trail

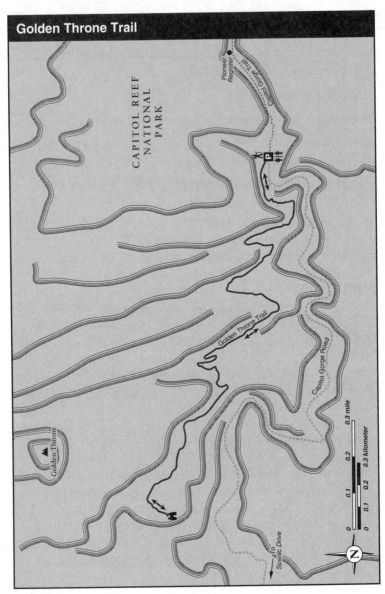

the trailhead, you'll see a large sign with metal letters on a sandstone block declaring an elevation gain of 1,100 vertical feet. It's a beautiful sign but, sadly, incorrect—the elevation gain is only about 700 feet.

From the parking area, the trail takes off to the left and ascends through a rocky section to backtrack along the road that brought you to the trailhead.

You'll be climbing steadily along ledges of Kayenta Formation and looking down to the wash below, on your left. It's always fun on an uphill trail to see your progress and how far you can ascend from the trailhead in just a few minutes. Very quickly you'll feel as though you're on top of the world after gaining just a few hundred feet.

The trail bends to the right, and you enter one of four deep-cut drainages that you'll circumvent along a mixed surface of slickrock and sandy sections. After rounding the first drainage and making your way back toward Capitol Gorge, you'll cross a flat section and soon enter a similar drainage. This pattern continues through the drainages until the Golden Throne comes into view on your right.

At the fourth flat section, you'll cross a slickrock grade where the route is marked by cairns. The Golden Throne occasionally disappears behind the closer cliffs but will suddenly reappear in your sights. Continuing for another 5 minutes, you'll ascend a small rise and reach the simple sign reading TRAIL'S END. At this point you can take in the views stretching to the Henry Mountains in the east and Golden Throne towering nearby. From the TRAIL'S END sign, make the short stroll to the south to gaze over the cliff and down to Scenic Drive and the Capitol Gorge Road before making your return to the trailhead.

TO THE TRAILHEAD
GPS Coordinates:
N38° 12.573' W111° 10.145'
From the Capitol Reef Visitor Center, drive south on Scenic Drive for 8.0 miles to the end of the pavement and the large picnic pavilion. Continue straight ahead at the junction on Capitol Gorge Road for 2.4 miles to the trailhead parking and picnic area.

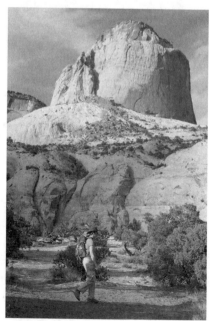

The Golden Throne

36 Chimney Rock Loop Trail

Trailhead Location: Chimney Rock Trailhead

Trail Use: Walking, hiking

Distance & Configuration: 3.5-mile balloon

Elevation Range: 6,060' at Chimney Rock Trailhead to 6,680' on the crest of the mesa

Facilities: Vault toilet at trailhead

Highlights: Panoramic views from the west side of Capitol Reef

DESCRIPTION

The trail's namesake is a stately pillar of rich red Moenkopi Formation that's clearly visible and best photographed from UT 24 near the trailhead. Chimney Rock is like a tower of puff pastry—hundreds of thin layers of sandstone sculpted by erosion and decoratively topped with a capstone of tan Shinarump Conglomerate. But once you're on the trail, Chimney Rock is largely out of view. What you'll see instead are Meeks Mesa and Chimney Rock Canyon, a small side canyon north of the mesa.

The mesa-top trail offers some commanding scenes in all directions, including the great barrier cliffs of Capitol Reef, the blackened plateaus of Boulder Mountain and Thousand Lakes Mountain to the west, and the Waterpocket Fold to the east.

Once on top of the mesa, you'll witness what becomes of a piñon–juniper woodland unprotected from the harsh winds of the desert—stunted specimens with gnarled and twisted trunks, and the wind-burnished remains of trees that never quite survived the buffeting of the elements.

ROUTE

From the trailhead parking area, the beaten path snakes northeast though Moenkopi mounds. Spring hikers can expect abundant desert wildflowers in addition to the piñon–juniper landscape. At 0.3 mile from the trailhead, you start ascending through the muted purple Chinle mounds along a series of steep, short switchbacks. With views of soaring Wingate Sandstone cliffs to the north, you gain most of your elevation through Chinle blocks, and at 0.5 mile you arrive at a junction sign directing you to the Chimney Rock Loop

Chimney Rock Loop Trail

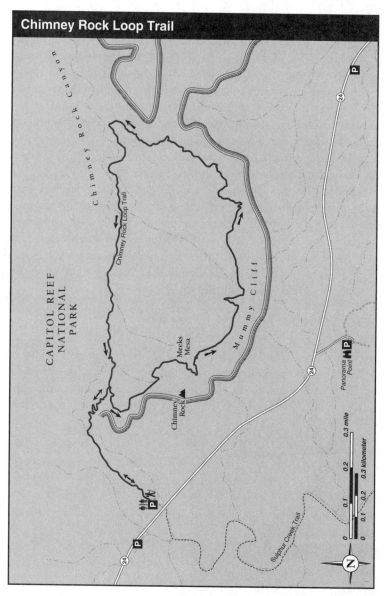

on the right. This marks the start of the counterclockwise loop and is where you'll return at the loop's completion.

The path continues climbing to reach the top of the mesa at 1.0 mile and soon comes to an overlook from the Mummy Cliff to Chimney Rock. In the distant west, you'll also see Boulder Mountain and Thousand Lakes

Mountain. While on the mesa, you'll have views of the reef and the Waterpocket Fold monocline to the east.

On your traverse of the mesa, you'll see the familiar piñons and junipers, but with a twist—literally—as the wind twists the wood of these century-old specimens. In the unforgiving mesa environment, you'll see hardy Mormon tea, but not much in the way of wildflowers or other delicate foliage. You'll also see the famous black boulders and wonder how they ever wound up on top of the mesa (see the opposite page for the answer).

At 1.2 miles, you'll begin your descent from Meeks Mesa onto an unnamed and less prominent mound to the east. The trail winds down to the north and goes into Chimney Rock Canyon. At 2.2 miles, you connect with the main canyon trail, almost completing the loop. In the canyon, the vegetation includes hopsage, desert trumpet, and rabbitbrush plants among the already familiar piñons, junipers, and Mormon tea shrubs. After you've crossed the sandy wash several times and made a slight ascent from the wash, you complete the loop by arriving back at the sign at 3.0 miles. From here, retrace your route to the trailhead.

TO THE TRAILHEAD
GPS Coordinates: N38° 18.938' W111° 18.234'
Enter Capitol Reef National Park on UT 24 from Torrey; the Chimney Rock Trailhead and parking area are 3.0 miles east of the park entrance sign and on your left. Alternatively, from the Capitol Reef Visitor Center, go 3.5 miles west on UT 24. The gravel trailhead parking area is on your right.

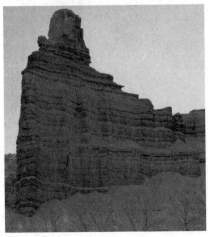

Chimney Rock

WHERE DID THOSE BLACK BOULDERS COME FROM?

As you're hiking around Capitol Reef, you will notice black basalt boulders of varying sizes in the unlikeliest of places—on top of mesas, along the river terraces, and resting on slickrock. Some of these boulders lie 500 feet or more above the elevation of the Fremont River. These boulders were produced in volcanic activity more than 20 million years ago. The boulders were then transported by flash floods, debris flows, and possibly glacial processes to their present locations. Large stones that differ from other rocks in the area and were carried by glaciers are called glacial erratics. But because similar black boulders are found through-out the area, including the nearby Boulder Mountain and Thousand Lakes Mountain, and because the rocks were not necessarily carried by glaciers, the term *glacial erratics* is an inaccurate descriptor of Capitol Reef's black boulders.

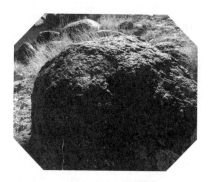

37 Sulphur Creek

Trailhead Location: Chimney Rock Trailhead

Trail Use: Walking, hiking

Distance & Configuration: 5.2-mile point-to-point

Elevation Range: 6,055' at Chimney Rock Trailhead to 5,520' at Capitol Reef Visitor Center parking lot

Facilities: Vault toilet at trailhead; restrooms and water at Capitol Reef Visitor Center

Highlights: A perennial stream carves its way through deep canyon narrows.

DESCRIPTION

Don't let the name fool you—Sulphur Creek is a crystal-clear perennial creek that has none of the brackish, cloudy, or odiferous qualities you might associate with sulfur. By the end of the hike you'll be playing and cooling yourself in this refreshing desert creek, a tributary of the Fremont River. Sulphur Creek is one of the most attractive slot canyons in Capitol Reef and a signature hike within a great hiking park.

The flow of the creek varies throughout the year based on rainfall, irrigation needs in Torrey, and snowmelt from its Thousand Lakes Mountain headwaters. But rarely will the water level be more than ankle-deep. Because there is no official trail—just the creek, which constricts through narrows and over small waterfalls—expect your feet to be wet much of the way, and come prepared with sandals, water shoes, or old sneakers.

You'll pass through the oldest exposed rocks in Capitol Reef on a hike that consists of four distinct segments: the dry wash from Chimney Rock to Sulphur Creek, the meandering creek bed, the narrows with its beautiful waterfalls, and the concluding stretch to the visitor center as the canyon again opens up and gives the creek some space to roam. Passing the three waterfalls requires traversing narrow ledges and down-climbing short sections. Though no technical gear (such as a rope or harness) is needed, there is some risk of falling, but never more than about 5 feet and usually into a pool of water just a few inches deep.

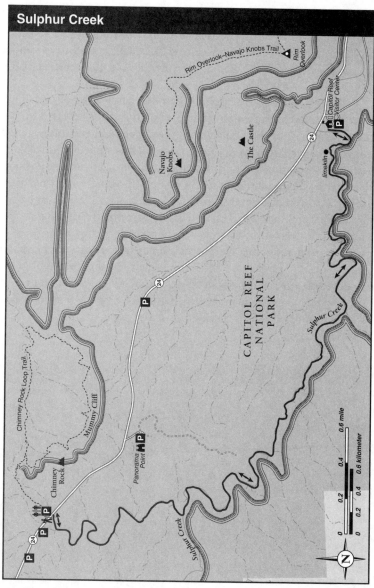

ROUTE

Sulphur Creek is ideally, and most frequently, hiked point-to-point, starting at the Chimney Rock Trailhead and concluding at the Capitol Reef
Visitor Center. Most visitors overcome this hurdle by leaving a shuttle

vehicle or bicycle at the visitor center. Alternatively, if you show up at the visitor center in need of a way back to Chimney Rock, you'll have little problem getting a ride. In fact, the ranger staff will even assist in connecting you with park visitors headed in that direction. In Capitol Reef, helping a fellow hiker is customary.

You'll access the route by crossing Utah 24 to the south side and dipping below the road level near a sign reading VISITOR CENTER VIA SULPHUR CREEK 5. Within 0.1 mile, you arrive at the larger wash and follow it down the canyon to your left. This dry wash continues its sinuous course along a sand-and-gravel bottom for 0.7 mile before arriving at a base layer of smooth rock. Soon the channel comes to a dry pour-off that can be easily negotiated on the left. At 1.5 miles from the trailhead, the dry wash arrives at Sulphur Creek, where you bear left and continue downstream. The rippling music of the creek will be your companion for the remainder of the route.

You'll need to cross the creek several times as you descend the canyon. Depending on the water level, this can normally be done without getting your feet wet. But as the canyon narrows, you might as well accept the fact that you're going to get wet. In fact, the park recommends that you hike in the wash bottom to avoid trampling the sparse plant communities on the dry banks.

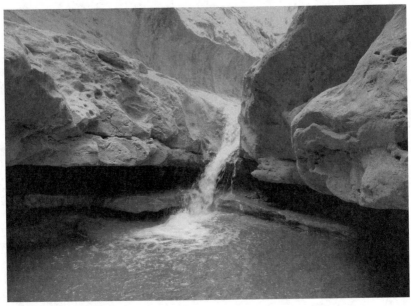

Waterfall in Sulphur Creek

Soon the canyon walls begin to close in and you enter the narrows, marked by a large log stuck between the two canyon walls. You'll most easily pass this first waterfall by down-climbing the ledges to your right. After a little more than 0.1 mile, you arrive at the second waterfall—no higher than the first but a little more difficult to pass. Your best route will be passing under a large rock on the right of the falls, and then descending three short pitches to the creek. You may find it easiest to take these descents sitting down.

If your feet aren't already wet, they will be as you now pass through the tightest section of the narrows. Before the canyon opens, you encounter one last waterfall, again most easily passable on the right.

As you approach the end of the route, you'll notice an old limekiln built by the early settlers of Fruita. Within 10 minutes and one final bend of the canyon, you'll be directly behind the visitor center, where you can ascend the slope on the right to enter the parking lot.

TO THE TRAILHEAD

GPS Coordinates: *Chimney Rock Trailhead:* N38º 18.938' W111º 18.234' *Capitol Reef Visitor Center:* N38º 17.474' W111º 15.770'
Enter the park on UT 24 from Torrey; the Chimney Rock Trailhead and parking area are 3.0 miles east of the park entrance sign and on your left. Alternatively, from the Capitol Reef Visitor Center, go 3.5 miles east on Utah 24. The gravel trailhead parking area is on your right. If you're doing this hike as a point-to-point, you will need to leave a vehicle at the visitor center or arrange for a shuttle.

WHY "CAPITOL REEF"?

Early visitors to the area thought that the various white domes of sandstone looked like the dome on the United States Capitol, thus giving this national park the first word in its name. The rocky cliffs were a major travel barrier, much like a coral reef is, resulting in the second word of the name. A similar use of the word *reef* has been applied to the San Rafael Reef to the northwest.

---

38 Rim Overlook

Trailhead Location: Rim Overlook

Trail Use: Walking, hiking

Distance & Configuration: 4.6-mile out-and-back

Elevation Range: 5,357' at trailhead to 6,375' at Rim Overlook

Facilities: Vault toilet at trailhead; no water

Highlights: Ascend from the Fremont River to an overlook with commanding views.

DESCRIPTION

Using the same riverside trailhead as the Hickman Bridge Trail (see page 131), you'll depart the shade and riparian vegetation to a cairn-marked slickrock route. The path leads to a spectacular overlook above sheer cliffs looking down into Fruita, Sulphur Creek, and the Fremont River Valley.

The Rim Overlook is the halfway stop on the longer Navajo Knobs Trail. And because it shares the same route of the Hickman Bridge Trail for the first 0.3 mile, it should be familiar territory for regular Capitol Reef hikers.

The cliffside setting of the overlook is not for the fainthearted. You're perched atop a sheer cliff with a 1,000-foot drop to the Fremont River

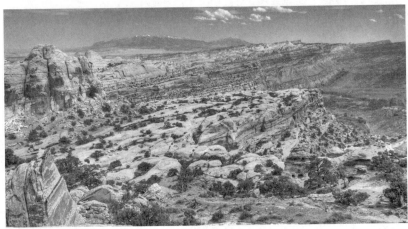

Capitol Reef National Park as seen from the Rim Overlook

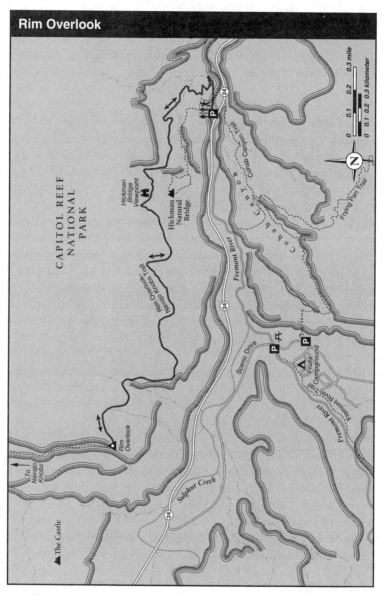

Rim Overlook

below. As if you were looking down from a hot-air balloon, you'll gaze at Fruita with its orchards, the Gifford house and barn, and the confluence of Sulphur Creek and the Fremont River.

Beyond the Waterpocket Fold to the east, the views include the Abajo Mountains and, in the far distance, the often-snowcapped Henry

Mountains. In the foreground you'll see the Navajo Domes, exposed by uplift and erosion and sculpted by the elements into magnificent buttes and pinnacles. To the south, Ferns Nipple is easily recognizable, and you can spot the switchbacks of the Cohab Canyon Trail.

ROUTE

From the Hickman Bridge Trailhead, follow the trail with the red Kayenta Formation cliffs on your left and the riparian vegetation of the Fremont River on your right. Even in the heat of summer, this short section is shaded and cooled by the nearby river flow. With a quick turn to the left, the path instantly departs the verdant riverbanks and ascends an arid, rocky, desert slope strewn with black volcanic boulders.

At 0.3 mile, you'll arrive at a signed junction where the path to the right directs you to the Rim Overlook–Navajo Knobs Trail, traveling among the distinctive black volcanic boulders found primarily in this part of the park. This junction is an ideal spot to face the east and view Capitol Dome, the park's namesake formation. From the junction, the trail ascends to the top of a ridge and then dips to cross a wash on slickrock. In addition to the black volcanic glacial erratics, you'll also see Moki marbles, iron oxide (hematite) balls that are produced in sandstone but are much harder and more resistant to erosion.

At 0.6 mile from the trailhead, the route departs from the wash and starts a switchbacked ascent to Hickman Bridge Viewpoint, at 0.8 mile. A stroll out to the ledge on the left of the sign gives you a lesser-seen view of one of Capitol Reef's most popular features.

From the viewpoint, the trail to the Rim Overlook ascends across flats and rises of Navajo Sandstone and winds its way into a series of four successive dry drainages. At the end of the fourth draw, you'll arrive at the sign for Rim Overlook, with the actual viewpoint to the left. If you're going on to the Navajo Knobs, the route lies straight ahead, but whether or not this is the turnaround point for your hike, you'll still want to take in the dizzying views from the cliff-top Rim Overlook before continuing on or returning to the trailhead.

TO THE TRAILHEAD

GPS Coordinates: N38º 17.325' W111º 13.656'
From the Capitol Reef Visitor Center, continue east on UT 24 for 2.0 miles. The trailhead parking area is on the north side of the road.

WHAT IS A MONOCLINE?

The Waterpocket Fold at Capitol Reef National Park is a great example of a monocline, which is a steplike fold or a wrinkle in the rock. All the layers in the rock, also known as strata, slope in the same direction. Imagine making a sandwich with layers of bread, meat, cheese, lettuce, and tomato, and then gently bending that sandwich in half; this gives you a pretty good visual picture of the earth's surface in a monocline.

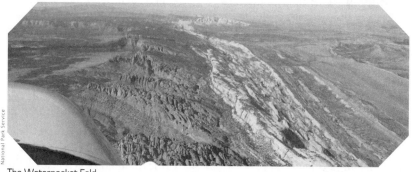

National Park Service

The Waterpocket Fold

39 Capitol Gorge Trail to The Tanks

Trailhead Location: Capitol Gorge Trailhead at the southern end of Scenic Drive

Trail Use: Walking, hiking

Distance & Configuration: 5.4-mile out-and-back

Elevation Range: 5,449' at Capitol Gorge Trailhead to 5,729' at The Tanks

Facilities: Vault toilet and covered picnic tables at trailhead; no water

Highlights: A walk along an old wagon trail to a cluster of potholes carved in stone—the defining geographic feature of Capitol Reef National Park, known as the Waterpocket Fold

DESCRIPTION

A stroll down the wash of Capitol Gorge takes you through one of only six drainages that cut through the Waterpocket Fold from east to west. This particular drainage was once a wagon road and subsequently a route used by motor vehicles before the construction of the present UT 24 in 1962. Capitol Gorge offered travelers a passage through the Waterpocket Fold that was free of the many Fremont River crossings required by the current UT 24 route.

The drive down Scenic Drive to the Capitol Gorge Trailhead is spectacular. Even if you don't have time for the hike, the drive to the trailhead alone is worth the time—if even for just a quick picnic in the shade of the pavilions. Along the way, don't hesitate to pull over, get out of your car, and take in the wonder.

Creating and maintaining the old road through Capitol Gorge was a demanding effort for the early settlers of the area. As prospectors and pioneers passed through the gorge, they carved their names on the rock walls, in a spot now known as the Pioneer Register.

In 1884, Elijah Cutler Behunin and several pioneer settlers struggled for eight days to clear boulders from a 3.5-mile stretch of Capitol Gorge. After they cleared the wash, two wagons—and later two cars—could pass one another. But their road through the Waterpocket Fold was short-lived. Eventually flash floods and rockfall returned the wash to its impassable, and often dangerous, natural state.

Capitol Gorge Trailhead to The Tanks

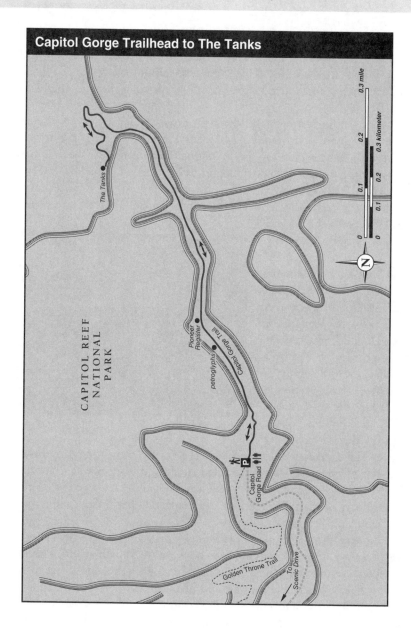

As the signs at the trailhead advise, always carry water with you when hiking in Capitol Reef, and in the confines of Capitol Gorge or other washes, beware of flash floods.

ROUTE

From the trailhead parking area, the trail stays above and to the left of the wash for the first 0.1 mile. Once you descend into the wash, you'll come to a weathered and scarred Fremont Indian petroglyph panel marked by a small pole.

The more interesting markings on the canyon wall begin about 100 yards past the Fremont petroglyphs, as early surveyors, prospectors, and travelers through the canyon chiseled inscriptions on the canyon wall. The first markings are the names of six surveyors from 1911.

As the canyon constricts you'll come to the Pioneer Register, where many of the early passersby left their inscriptions. The earliest are from 1871, when JA CALL and WAL. BATEMAN, two early prospectors in search of gold, put their names on the wall. Iron poles protruding from the canyon walls are the remains of a telephone line that was strung through the canyon in the early 20th century.

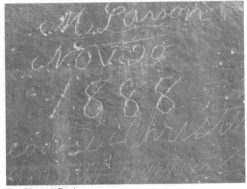

The Pioneer Register

At 0.8 mile from the trailhead, the wash opens a bit, and you'll come to a sign on the left directing you to The Tanks at 0.2 mile. From the sign, the trail ascends through a jumble of boulders with unexpected twists and turns marked by cairns. After making a quick climb, the trail levels out and you arrive at a junction where the most distinctive feature is a manzanita bush. Continuing on to the right, you arrive at The Tanks.

Some of the water pockets are filled with water only in the spring or after a heavy rainstorm, but the larger ones always contain water. Additionally, they are teeming with the larvae of many species, including insects and frogs. Exploring the area around The Tanks, you'll also find a small natural bridge with a few other potholes normally filled with water. All of these potholes are essential sources of water for wildlife in the area, as well as a micro-ecosystem for the plant and animal life within each pothole. Once you've discovered and explored The Tanks, return to the trailhead along the same path.

TO THE TRAILHEAD

GPS Coordinates: N38º 12.573' W111º 10.145'

From the Capitol Reef Visitor Center, drive south on Scenic Drive for 8.0 miles to the end of the pavement and to the large picnic pavilion. At the junction, continue straight ahead on Capitol Gorge Road for 2.4 miles to the trailhead parking and picnic area.

LIFE IN THE POTHOLES

Potholes, known to early visitors as water pockets, are geologic depressions in bedrock that resemble the holes found in Swiss cheese. The water you see in the potholes comes directly from precipitation. If you look closely at some of these pockets, especially the larger ones, you may see something unexpected: many of them are teeming with life. Bacteria, diatoms, algae, and fungi abound in these small ecosystems. Some of the potholes contain rare, ancient organisms that are not found elsewhere.

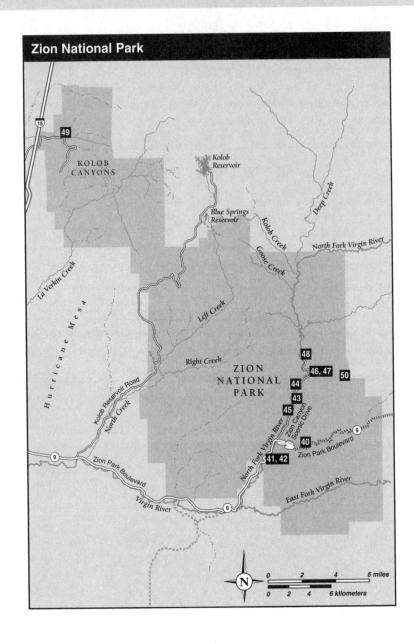

Zion National Park

ZION NATIONAL PARK

Park Overview

With more than 2 million visitors per year, Zion is Utah's most heavily visited national park. Its glowing sandstone cliffs, towering cathedrals, and lush fern-clad sanctuaries offer visitors a stunningly beautiful setting. With dozens of wet and dry slot canyons, more big-wall climbing routes than Yosemite, a mild climate, and hundreds of miles of hiking trails, Zion is a mecca for adventure seekers. There's something for everyone in Zion, and 70% of Zion's visitors take a hike on the park's trails.

The dramatic centerpiece of the park is Zion Canyon, a 15-mile-long and up to 0.5-mile-deep slice through Navajo Sandstone cut by the North Fork of the Virgin River. From the canyon floor to the summit of Horse Ranch Mountain, there is more than 5,000 feet of elevation differential, which produces an array of eco-zones and an abundant variety of plant and animal species. Zion's hospitable climate and agriculturally productive river terraces have hosted humans for more than 8,000 years.

Utah's oldest national park was established in 1909 as Mukuntuweap National Monument. In 1918, the acting director of the newly created National Park Service observed that the name was too hard to pronounce and remember. So the name was changed to Zion, and a year later it became America's 12th national park.

JUST ONE DAY?

Zion handles its crowds efficiently with a shuttle system that operates April–October and connects the town of Springdale and the park visitor center with Zion Canyon, as well as all of the popular sites and trailheads. After a stop at the visitor center, board the shuttle bound for Zion Canyon. If you're ready for a strenuous climb, visit The Grotto and make a morning ascent of Angels Landing. Those looking for a gentler excursion can instead hike the Emerald Pools Trail at Zion Lodge. Continuing on up the canyon, stop at Weeping Rock for the short path to this natural seep in the sandstone. Conclude your day at the Temple of Sinawava, where you can enjoy the Riverside Walk as it begins its entry into the Narrows of the Virgin River.

If you're arriving in Zion from US 89 and Mt. Carmel Junction on the east, make your first stop just before entering the tunnel to hike the Canyon Overlook Trail for a sneak peek at Zion Canyon.

◘ ◘ ◘

40 Canyon Overlook Trail

Trailhead Location: On the north side of UT 9, immediately east of the Mt. Carmel Tunnel

Trail Use: Walking, hiking

Distance & Configuration: 1.0-mile out-and-back

Elevation Range: 5,147' at trailhead to 5,310' at the Canyon Overlook

Facilities: Restrooms at trailhead parking area

Highlights: A short but exciting trail to a dramatic overlook

DESCRIPTION

The Canyon Overlook Trail packs a lot of adventure into 1 mile and culminates in a dramatic overlook, with Pine Creek Canyon in the foreground and Zion Canyon beyond. Built by the Civilian Conservation Corps in the early 1930s, the path reflects the trail-building craftsmanship found in other national parks of the same era, such as Grand Canyon and Yosemite. You'll find some steep drop-offs along the route, but the terrain and short distance make it great for hikers of varied abilities, though you'll want to keep young children close at hand.

If you're entering Zion National Park from the east, this would be an excellent first hike before proceeding through the Mt. Carmel Tunnel and spending the remainder of your stay in and around Zion Canyon. The trail and overlook are also a wonderful way to whet your appetite and give you a sneak peek of the majesty that awaits.

ROUTE

On a busy weekend, the most challenging part of this hike might be finding a parking place, and the most dangerous part could be crossing UT 9, which bisects the park east to west, to access the trailhead on the north side of the road, so use the crosswalk. Once you've successfully accomplished those two feats, you'll discover that the Canyon Overlook Trail has more personality per square inch than any other hike in the park. Given its lofty setting and varied terrain, you'll want to avoid this hike in the rain or if lightning is present.

Canyon Overlook Trail

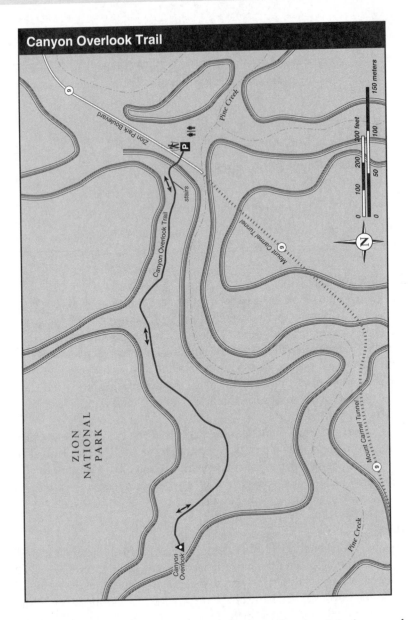

The route begins by quickly departing the trailhead and the busy roadway via a sandstone stairway, where most of the hike's elevation gain is earned. The trail is well maintained and supplied with handrails and fencing, when needed, to provide extra protection.

You'll be treated to an abundant variety of trailside trees, shrubs, and wildflowers for such a short hike. Utah juniper, shrub live oak, and single-leaf ash mix with piñon, mountain mahogany, and Utah serviceberry.

Hoodoos, sculpted cliffs, and weathered boulders add visual appeal to the winding route through Pine Creek Canyon on a mixed trail surface of slickrock, sand, and compacted dirt. With a bend to the right, the trail enters a classic Zion alcove, similar to others in Zion Canyon, adorned with maidenhair ferns, indicative of the perennial moisture seeping through fissures in the sandstone. The alcove offers some of the only shade on the trail, so if you're hiking in the midday sun, you'll enjoy the cooling respite.

Emerging from the alcove and passing a pile of rock that has fallen from the cliffs above, you'll soon arrive at the end of the trail. From the edge of the cliff, thankfully protected by a sturdy railing and chain-link fence, you'll overlook Pine Creek Canyon with the lower portion of Zion Canyon in the distance. The overlook offers fine views of the Beehives, West Temple, and East Temple—all prominent features of Zion National Park.

Among all the natural wonders, be sure to take note of the park's most notable man-made wonder, the Zion–Mt. Carmel Tunnel. From the overlook, you can see where waste rock from the tunnel construction was dumped into Pine Creek Canyon below. Great photo opportunities abound at the cliffside overlook, and you'll enjoy playing on the surrounding rock formations before making your return.

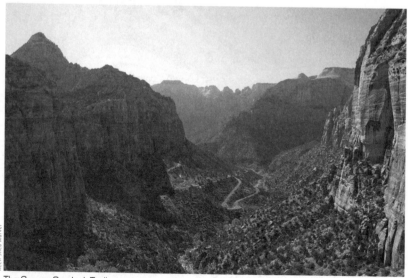

The Canyon Overlook Trail

TO THE TRAILHEAD

GPS Coordinates: N37º 12.802' W112º 56.443'

From the Zion National Park entrance in Springdale, take UT 9 east toward the Zion–Mt. Carmel Tunnel. Immediately after exiting the tunnel, make a right into the trailhead parking lot. If this parking lot is full, additional parking is about 100 yards farther down the road, on the left.

THE ZION–MT. CARMEL TUNNEL

Cut through 1.1 miles of solid sandstone, the Zion–Mt. Carmel Tunnel first connected the east side of the park with Zion Canyon and Springdale in 1930. Started in 1927 and built at a cost of $1.9 million

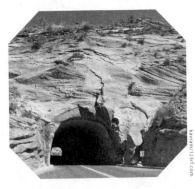

(including the highway), it was the longest tunnel in the United States when it was completed. It required 292,320 pounds of dynamite to build the tunnel and road. At its dedication ceremony, then–Utah Governor George Dern declared that it was "the most remarkable road ever built."

Before the tunnel was completed, the only way to access Zion Canyon was from Springdale on the west. But the lure of tourism revenue and the popularity of the Union Pacific's Grand Circle Tour bus route, which included Zion, the Grand Canyon, and Bryce Canyon, made easy access from the east especially desirable.

41 Pa'rus Trail

Trailhead Location: On the east side of the Zion Canyon Visitor Center, near the shuttle terminal

Trail Use: Walking, hiking, cycling, wheelchair-accessible, leashed pets

Distance & Configuration: 7.0-mile out-and-back or 3.5-mile point-to-point

Elevation Range: 3,918' at Zion Canyon Visitor Center trailhead to 4,030' at the Canyon Junction shuttle stop

Facilities: Water, restrooms, and picnic tables at Zion Canyon Visitor Center and in South Campground

Highlights: Riverside walk connecting visitor center with South Campground and Zion Canyon

DESCRIPTION

The Pa'rus Trail is a popular multi-use trail that winds alongside and crosses the Virgin River between the visitor center and Canyon Junction at the mouth of Zion Canyon. The name *Pa'rus* comes from a Paiute word meaning "bubbling, tumbling water," and the relaxing gurgle of the river is nearby throughout this hike. In addition to the river, you'll find good bird-watching in the dense riverbank vegetation, as well as numerous opportunities to access the river.

This may be the ideal early-morning walk in Zion, and one that everybody can enjoy. If you are staying in the adjacent campground, then nothing could be

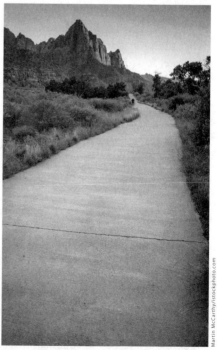

Pa'rus Trail with The Watchman in the distance

more convenient, and you'll be using the Pa'rus Trail as you walk to the visitor center or into Springdale for groceries or shopping. The trail is paved and at least 10 feet wide throughout, so there's enough room to walk or run, ride a bicycle, or push a stroller. And for those using a wheelchair, Pa'rus is the most accessible trail in the park. It's also a very sociable trail, where families and couples take time to greet one another in passing and even stop for a friendly chat.

ROUTE

Most visits to Zion National Park begin at the visitor center, a spacious complex with ample parking, easily accessed from Springdale by park shuttle, by car, or on foot. With its theater, interpretive displays both inside and outside, and park rangers to help you map out your visit, you should be well prepared as you make your way to the shuttle stop in front of the visitor center. The Pa'rus Trailhead is across the Virgin River, over the bridge, and about 100 feet north of the shuttle stop.

For the first 0.5 mile, the trail gently follows the riverbank to the right, with South Campground to the left. You'll have many opportunities to wade in the river, so don't hesitate to take off your shoes, play in the water, and be a kid again. Just be sure to use the designated river access points rather than risk damaging biological soil crusts or revegetation areas.

After leaving the campground and crossing an access road, you come to your first bridge crossing—not over the Virgin, but a small side-canyon tributary. At 0.6 mile from the trailhead, you'll see an unpaved spur to the left leading to the Zion Human History Museum, which showcases American Indian culture, pioneer settlement, and Zion's growth as a national park.

At 0.8 mile from the trailhead, you'll come to the first of several sturdy bridges crossing both the Virgin River and side-canyon tributaries. While walking over one of the bridges, observe the course of the river and consider that this river, as well as flow from other smaller side canyons, was instrumental in carving the immense canyons that lay before you. The flow of the Virgin River fluctuates widely throughout the year depending on rain, snowmelt, and air temperatures. And because the Zion backcountry is so popular with hikers and canyoneers, the park monitors Virgin River flows continually as a means of gauging safety conditions in The Narrows of the Virgin River and other side canyons.

You'll cross the river three times and Pine Creek once as you ascend the canyon at an almost imperceptible grade. Over the course of 3.5 miles, you gain only 112 feet of elevation, allowing you to save your energy for some of the more aerobic hikes in Zion Canyon—of which there are plenty. Shortly

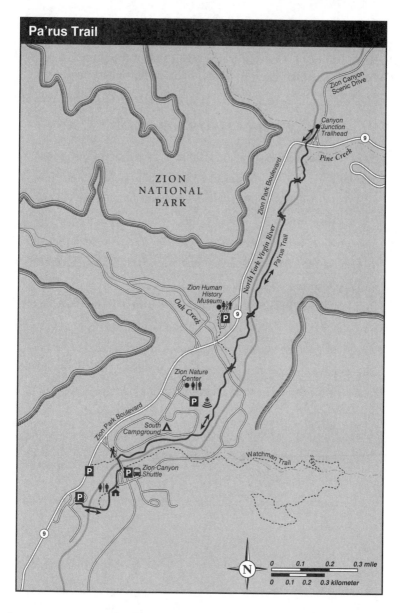

Pa'rus Trail

after crossing the Pine Creek bridge, the path dips and crosses under UT 9; it then makes a short ascent to arrive at the Canyon Junction shuttle stop and the end of the trail. From here, the shuttle can return you to the visitor center or take you for an onward trip up Zion Canyon.

TO THE TRAILHEAD

GPS Coordinates: N37º 12.110' W112º 59.203'

The Pa'rus Trailhead is located on the north side of the Virgin River, about 100 feet from the Zion Canyon Visitor Center shuttle terminal.

ZION CANYON SHUTTLE

Back in 1997, with 2.4 million visitors per year, Zion Canyon was regularly congested with cars. Parking was a hassle, and protecting vegetation, wildlife habitat, and the treasured tranquility of the canyon were real concerns. The shuttle system established in 2000 now provides visitors with a relaxing, efficient, and eco-friendly way to visit the park. Private vehicle traffic is restricted March–October in Zion Canyon.

Today, 75% of Zion's annual visitors use the shuttle, which saves more than 50,000 vehicle miles per day and reduces CO_2 emissions by more than 12 tons per day. One unexpected benefit of the system is that Zion has now become a bicycle-friendly park, with many visitors bringing their bikes (or renting bikes in Springdale) and enjoying the splendor of Zion Canyon on a two-wheeler. The buses are equipped with a front rack and can carry two bicycles, so you can ride your bike as much as you want and still get some motorized assistance if needed.

42 Watchman Trail

Trailhead Location: Across the street from the Zion Canyon Visitor Center shuttle terminal

Trail Use: Walking, hiking

Distance & Configuration: 3.2-mile balloon

Elevation Range: 3,910' at Zion Canyon Visitor Center trailhead to 4,287' at viewpoint

Facilities: Water and restrooms at Zion Canyon Visitor Center

Highlights: From the banks of the Virgin River to a plateau with impressive views of the canyon floor and some of Zion's mountain cathedrals

DESCRIPTION

Though not a showpiece or destination hike, the Watchman Trail, with its trailhead near the Zion Canyon Visitor Center, is a great early-morning leg

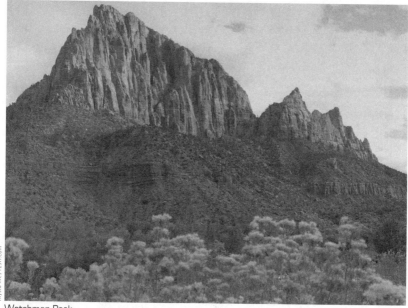

Alysta Inc./123rf.com

Watchman Peak

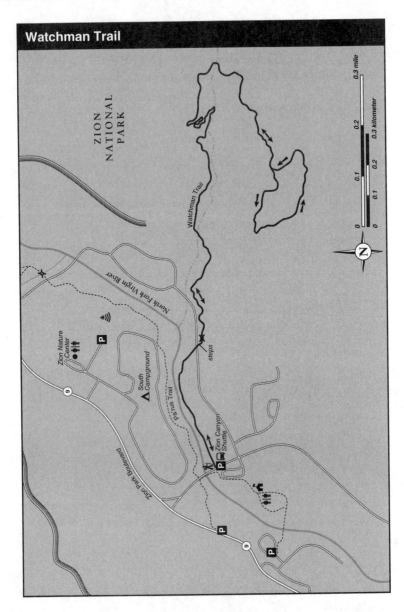

stretcher—easily accessible from the Watchman Campground and from many of the accommodations in Springdale. It's a varied route with a mix of riparian and desert vegetation; it also takes you from an alluvial outwash, through a steep-walled canyon, and onto a red-rock desert bench.

The Watchman Formation, which lends its name to this trail and to the park's main campground, is the symmetrical and ribbed red spire just to the south of the park entrance.

Wide, well marked, and well maintained, this trail is suitable for hikers of all skill levels. The path offers little shade, so be sure to reserve this hike for early morning or late afternoon.

ROUTE

The Watchman Trail begins just across the road from the Zion Canyon shuttle terminal. Use the crosswalk to access the dirt trail on the south side of the Virgin River, where an interpretive sign and map mark the trailhead. The trail follows the contour of the riverbank for the first 0.25 mile before crossing the park-residence access road.

Immediately upon crossing the access road, you'll notice that the vegetation changes from a riparian setting dominated by Fremont cottonwoods to a desert canyon dotted with single-leaf piñons and Utah junipers. The trail ascends steps of sandstone blocks and crosses a sturdy wooden bridge. To your left, note the park-employee residences on the canyon floor below.

After crossing this bench, the trail enters a scenic side canyon with cliffs of Springdale Sandstone, a hard layer with sturdy cliffs set on top of the softer Moenave Formation, resulting in overhangs and eroded slopes. The slopes are dotted with large angular blocks of reddish sandstone that have fallen from the cliffs above, which, after falling, are exposed to weathering and split in two, looking as if they were neatly cut by a giant butcher knife.

Continuing up the canyon, the trail ascends rapidly via four neatly carved switchbacks. After hiking about 1 mile from the trailhead, you'll pass several small seeps that trickle across slabs of sandstone on the trail and bestow a lushness to the canyon expressed in cottonwoods, ferns, box elders, and seasonal wildflowers. Throughout the canyon you'll also see yucca bushes, beavertail cacti, and other members of the piñon–juniper woodland, such as single-leaf ash, buffaloberry, and Utah serviceberry.

At 1.3 miles the trail emerges onto a spacious bench with impressive views to the north, west, and south. Here, the path forks and the sign directs you to the right as you begin a scenic 0.4-mile loop that will return you to this spot. The loop begins with a gentle descent and soon offers a worthwhile spur on the right that leads in just 100 feet to an admirable overlook at an elevation of 4,420 feet. Spread out below and to the northwest is Springdale, a Mormon settlement dating to 1860 and now the gateway community to the park, which accommodates most of Zion's 2.6 million annual visitors.

Many of Zion's iconic towers, including the Towers of the Virgin (with its vertical relief of nearly 4,000 feet) and the West Temple, lie to the north. Continuing on this loop, you'll soon make a gentle ascent that will return you to the fork and enable you to retrace your route back to the trailhead.

TO THE TRAILHEAD

GPS Coordinates: N37° 12.082' W112° 59.185'

From the Zion Canyon Visitor Center shuttle terminal, cross the street to the marked trailhead. The trail can also be accessed from the Watchman Campground.

PIÑON PINES

Piñon (or pinyon) pines are a group of eight different conifers whose cones yield edible piñon nuts. These trees are found throughout the Southwest and in each of the five national parks in Utah. The most common species within Zion National Park is the single-leaf piñon—easy to identify because most pine trees have two-, three-, or five-needle clusters, but as its name suggests, the single-leaf piñon does not have clustered needles.

Piñon nuts, or pine nuts as they're popularly called, were a staple of the American Indian diet. High in nutrients and an especially good source of monounsaturated fatty acids, pine nuts are frequently sprinkled on salads or baked in bread, and they are essential ingredients in Italian pesto.

Piñon pines also serve as a food source for some animal species in the Southwest. The nuts are an important part of the diet of the piñon jay, a bird that is essential to the regeneration of piñon woodlands. Piñon jays store thousands of seeds during the year, and while they return to find and eat many of them, they also leave many in the ground, which then sprout and grow into new trees.

43 Emerald Pools Trail

Trailhead Location: In Zion Canyon at the ?

Trail Use: Walking, hiking

Distance & Configuration: 1.3-mile out-and-back to Lower Pool or 2.2-mile out-and-back to Upper Pool; can be hiked as an out-and-back or loop with connecting options to other park trails

Elevation Range: 4,277' at Zion Lodge shuttle stop to 4,680' at Upper Emerald Pool

Facilities: Water, restrooms, restaurants, and full facilities at Zion Lodge

Highlights: A fun and varied network of trails leading to the beautiful alcoves, waterfalls, and pools of Zion Canyon

DESCRIPTION

The Emerald Pools Trails are among the most popular hiking trails in the park, and justifiably so. From the valley floor, the trail crosses the Virgin River and ascends through three sets of pools. The route passes through varied habitats: riparian, desert, and cool canyon—each with its own microhabitats. Along the way, you'll have panoramic views up and down the canyon before entering deeply set alcoves.

Perennial seeps in the sandstone feed the pools, and seasonal runoff from the rim augments them. So the water flow, ranging from a trickle to gushing waterfalls, keeps the pools filled with water year-round and creates microhabitats for a wide variety of plants and animals. The emerald hue surrounding the pools, especially the Upper and Lower

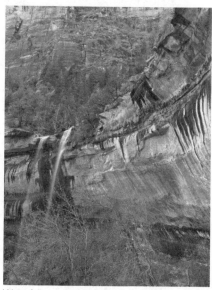

Waterfalls pour over a cliff at Lower Emerald Pools.

Colin D. Young/ilightphoto/istockphoto.com

Emerald Pools Trail

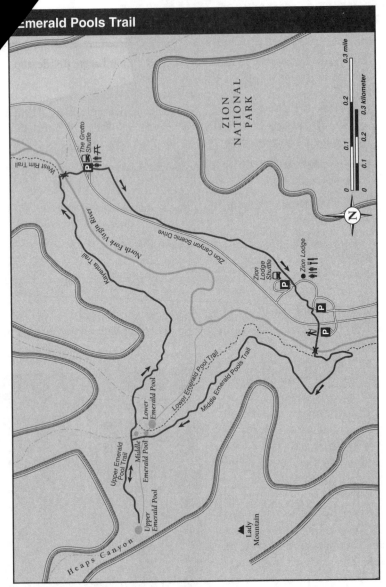

Pools, is primarily from algae, but maidenhair ferns and lush vegetation complement the green palette.

With three pools from which to choose—Upper, Middle, and Lower— you have several options for how you tackle these trails, which pools you visit, and which onward and connecting trails you follow. With all the signage and natural topography of the canyon, getting lost is virtually impossible, but getting separated from hiking companions can happen very easily and quickly, so pay attention and have a prearranged meeting spot, such as Zion Lodge, at the end of your hike.

On a hot summer day, the trail offers abundant shade and a cooling spray from the seeps, but please don't swim or wade in the pools.

ROUTE

Zion Lodge is the closest shuttle stop to this hike and also offers the best-equipped trailhead in the park, with water, restrooms, trail snacks, and dining options. From the large, grassy area in front of the lodge, cross Zion Canyon Scenic Drive and walk in the direction of the sturdy footbridge that crosses the Virgin River. Once across the bridge, you'll come to a sign directing you to the Lower Pool at 0.6 mile, the Middle Pool at 0.9 mile, and the Upper Pool at 1.2 miles.

A gently ascending paved pitch parallels the Virgin River on your right, with the flanks of Lady Mountain to your left; you'll continue for 0.25 mile before bending to the left as the trail makes its entry into Heaps Canyon. Here you're treated to a mixed-forest canopy of Fremont cottonwoods, Gambel oaks, box elders, bigtooth maples, and junipers. The sounds of canyon birds accompany you throughout the trail and especially in this forested section.

At just beyond 0.5 mile after the bridge over the Virgin River, you arrive at the Lower Pool, set within an immense alcove festooned with moss and ferns. The fragmented and polished concrete trail surface loops the alcove and has a handrail for added safety as you occasionally dodge sprays of water from above.

Ascending beyond the Lower Pool for just 0.1 mile, you come to a junction with a sign pointing to the Middle Pool. Take a hard left and make a steep ascent through boulders and on steps made from large sandstone blocks, soon passing through a cleft between two cabin-size sandstone blocks.

Arriving at the Middle Pool, you're on a slickrock sandstone slab where pools have formed by water trickling from above. To your left is a drop-off that drains down to the Lower Pool. Cross the Middle Pool slab and find a trail making its way up and to the right, where you'll see a landing with benches and a sign that directs you to Upper Emerald Pool at 0.3 mile.

As it approaches the Upper Pool, the trail ascends steeply, winding its way through a jumble of boulders before making a short descent into the basin containing the pool. You have some return options, which include returning the way you came. But for a little variety, consider taking the

Kayenta Trail from the junction below the Middle Pool to the Grotto shuttle stop (an additional 1.0 mile), where you can continue up the canyon on the shuttle or return to Zion Lodge by way of the Grotto Trail (an additional 0.6 mile).

TO THE TRAILHEAD

GPS Coordinates: N37º 15.057' W112º 57.439'
Take the Zion shuttle to the Zion Lodge shuttle stop. In the off-season (November–late March), when the shuttle is not in operation, drive from Canyon Junction (the junction of UT 9 and Zion Canyon Scenic Drive) north on Zion Canyon Scenic Drive for 2.6 miles to the parking area, on the left side of the road.

KANGAROO RATS

This amazing rodent is highly adapted to living in the desert. Kangaroo rats have complex burrow systems that are used to store food, escape predators, and shelter them from the summer heat. Their tails are longer than their bodies and heads combined. This long tail is useful for stability; some species of kangaroo rat have been known to travel 7–8 feet in one leap and can even change directions in midair! Kangaroo rats use random zigzagging flight patterns to avoid becoming prey. The rodents also have breakaway tails—when a predator grabs the tuft at the end of their tail, that part will break off and regrow.

Their fur color also helps them survive. It blends in extremely well with the surrounding dirt and rocks, so it's possible to overlook a kangaroo rat right by you. Kangaroo rats can live their entire lives without taking a sip of water because they get all the water they need from their food. In addition, their nasal passages collect water from each outgoing breath to help keep them hydrated.

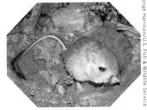
George Harrison/U.S. Fish & Wildlife Service

44 Angels Landing

Trailhead Location: In Zion Canyon at the Grotto shuttle stop

Trail Use: Walking, hiking

Distance & Configuration: 5.2-mile out-and-back

Elevation Range: 4,279' at the Grotto shuttle stop to 5,990' at the Angels Landing summit

Facilities: Restrooms, water, and picnic area at the Grotto shuttle stop

Highlights: A thrilling and challenging hike with steep drop-offs and spectacular mountaintop views

DESCRIPTION

One of the signature hikes in Zion National Park, and one of the very best short hikes in the United States, takes the West Rim Trail from The Grotto picnic area to Angels Landing. The climb to the top takes on the characteristics of a heroic journey as you overcome a series of obstacles. Along the way you'll traverse and surmount iconic features with legendary names, such as Refrigerator Canyon, Walter's Wiggles, Scout Lookout, and the Step of Faith. The trek culminates in a slickrock stroll to the crest of Angels Landing.

Built in 1926, the trail to Angels Landing was among the first in the park. The section of tight switchbacks known as Walter's Wiggles is an engineering marvel, an exquisitely sculpted route up a cliff to the Scout Lookout viewpoint, with Angels Landing another 0.5 mile beyond.

Those who complete the hike deserve bragging rights, because not all who start this trail finish. They turn back—and they should—when at any point they feel uncomfortable, at risk, or in danger. Be advised that the final section includes a steep, narrow ridge to the summit, and at some points the trail is no more than 3 feet wide, with 1,000-foot drop-offs on either side. It's not for the fainthearted or anyone afraid of heights, and it's not recommended for young children.

Since the trail opened in 1926, no fewer than nine people have fallen to their deaths on Angels Landing. Avoid the trail any time compacted snow or ice is on the route, and steer clear of Angels Landing during rain or when there is a chance of lightning. Even in perfect conditions, there are sections of the trail where you'll need to grab on to chains with both hands and step very carefully.

But for prepared hikers on a clear day, this rewarding hike concludes with you standing on the top of this sentinel monolith. The views from Angels Landing are some of the best in the park, and the hike will provide you with memories for years to come.

ROUTE

Fill your water bottles at the Grotto parking area and shuttle stop, and then cross Zion Canyon Scenic Drive in the direction of the Virgin River. At 0.1 mile, walk across the river on a sturdy footbridge. At the end of the bridge, turn right on a signed trail that shows Scout Lookout at 2.0 miles and Angels Landing at 2.5 miles.

The paved route initially leads north, with the Virgin River on your right, and then rises on switchbacks to the cooling depths of Refrigerator Canyon, a narrow chasm with the Navajo Sandstone walls of Angels Landing on your right.

It's a steady but fairly gentle ascent up Refrigerator Canyon before the trail reverses itself and enters the 21 tight switchbacks that constitute Walter's Wiggles. Once at the top of the switchbacks, you emerge onto Scout Lookout, a sandy landing dotted with ponderosa pines that also serves as the junction of the West Rim Trail, which enters from the north. For

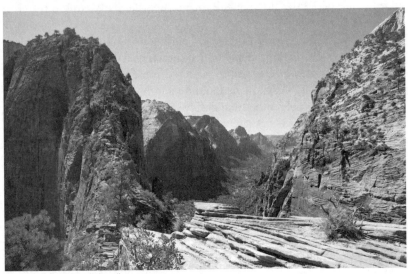

Near the top of Angels Landing

Angels Landing

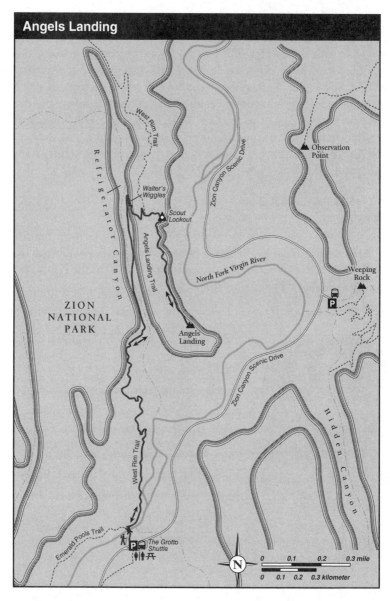

many, Scout Lookout is the end of the Angels Landing hike, and they will be nicely rewarded with some fine views. But for more-serious hikers, the summit of Angels Landing is just 0.5 mile ahead.

The onward route to Angels Landing starts gently enough through pines on a wide path. Then you come to the north ridge of the landing, where a narrow sandstone rib defines the rocky route. Steps have been carefully cut into the stable and secure rock face, but you can't avoid gazing down cliffs with sheer drops of 500 feet or more. One of these steps, known as the Step of Faith, is a sandstone block with a step cut in the center. On the right side is the chain railing, and on the left is a sheer drop. You'll want to keep a steady hand on the chain. Nearing the top among ponderosa pines, the trail leads to the crest of Angels Landing, with commanding views into the canyon below and an easy gaze eastward across the canyon to the Great White Throne. Enjoy the scenery and a snack before carefully making your way back—downhill all the way.

TO THE TRAILHEAD

GPS Coordinates: N37º 15.597' W112º 57.088'

From the Zion Canyon Visitor Center, take the Zion Canyon Shuttle to the Grotto shuttle stop. November–March, enter Zion National Park by car and take Zion Canyon Scenic Drive north for 3.4 miles to the Grotto picnic area, where you'll find ample parking.

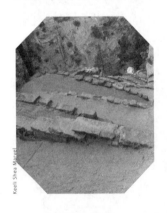

BUILDING WALTER'S WIGGLES

The 21 switchbacks you see on the way to Angels Landing were constructed in 1926 and named after the park's first custodian and superintendent, Walter Reusch. This trail is known as one of the most dramatic routes ever built by the National Park Service. The "wiggles" help prevent erosion on the path. Can you imagine the courage and tenacity it must have taken for workers to chisel out by hand the first footholds in this trail?

45 Court of the Patriarchs

Trailhead Location: In Zion Canyon at the Court of the Patriarchs shuttle stop

Trail Use: Walking, hiking; also horse tours

Distance & Configuration: 1.4-mile point-to-point

Elevation Range: 4,266' at Court of the Patriarchs shuttle stop to 4,350' on a knoll above the river

Facilities: No water or restrooms at the trailhead or on trail; water, restrooms, restaurants, and full facilities at Zion Lodge at trail's end

Highlights: Enter Zion Canyon on foot in the shadows of the Patriarchs.

DESCRIPTION

The Court of the Patriarchs is the first shuttle stop after you enter Zion Canyon and begin the dramatic ascent. Most visitors stay on the bus and glance at the three Patriarchs from the shuttle's windows. But if you have a few days to enjoy the park and aren't rushed, then stopping at Court of the Patriarchs and leisurely walking to Zion Lodge is a wonderful way to enter the heart of the canyon—evoking the days when early settlers walked the riverbanks and gazed in amazement at the towering mountain cathedrals above.

Those pioneering explorations of Zion Canyon must have been thrilling outings. Early visitors were seemingly so inspired by the towers within Zion Canyon that they gave the mountains names such as the Great White Throne, Angels Landing, Mountain of the Sun, and the Altar of Sacrifice. Some of the first towers they would have encountered are three similarly shaped white-topped pinnacles, which they named after the biblical patriarchs Abraham, Isaac, and Jacob (west to east). This cluster of peaks is collectively known as the Court of the Patriarchs.

The Court of the Patriarchs Trail is the shortest route in Zion National Park—a 150-foot paved path that quickly snakes up the hillside. At the top is a lookout point with views you won't want to miss and a perspective that makes for a perfect photo every time.

After ascending to the Court of the Patriarchs overlook, cross the street and follow the Emerald Pools Trail Connector along the Virgin River to Zion Lodge.

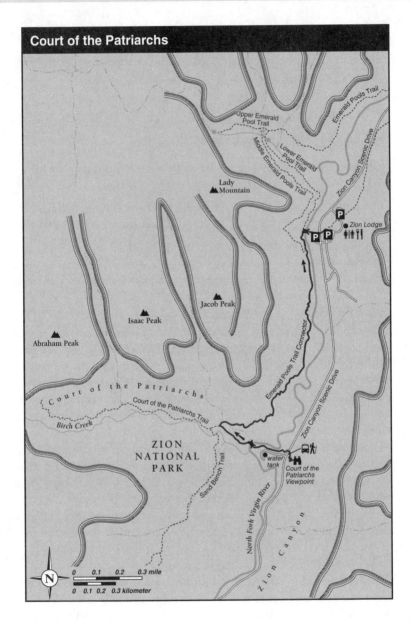

Court of the Patriarchs

ROUTE

Arriving at the Court of the Patriarchs shuttle stop, get off the shuttle and make the quick jaunt up to the Court of the Patriarchs viewpoint. It's just 150 feet to the observation landing along the steep, paved trail, and you'll be there in just a few minutes. From this overlook you'll have perfectly framed vistas of the Court of the Patriarchs—Abraham Peak, Isaac Peak, and Jacob Peak—so have your camera ready. Returning to the bus stop, you can take the next bus up the canyon to Zion Lodge, or you can follow the route described here and walk just over a mile to the lodge, capturing some even closer views of the Patriarchs and strolling along a gentle riverside trail.

From the shuttle stop, cross Zion Canyon Scenic Drive to the west and walk onto the unmarked trail leading to the west, with the service road on your left and the Virgin River on your right. Walk 0.1 mile to a footbridge crossing the Virgin River. At the end of the bridge, after crossing the river, turn right and continue up a small rise leading in the direction of the Court of the Patriarchs. At the top of this rise, about 0.2 mile from the shuttle stop, you'll have a dazzling up close view of the Patriarchs, towering directly in front of you—almost too close to photograph. From this mound, you'll look down and see the wooden fences of the horse trail.

Continue along the trail as it descends toward the fences. Arriving at an unsigned junction, turn right. Turning left will put you on the Sand Bench Loop, a sandy horse trail that makes for an unpleasant foot trail. Take the trail to your right, which is the northern extension of the Sand Bench Trail, also known as the Emerald Pools Trail Connector; it's used by horses, but it's a better, more suitable surface for hiking than the Sand Bench Trail. This trail drops into a small side canyon, stays below the bench on your left, and offers some shade. Soon the trail bends to the left and, while staying at a low elevation, starts to parallel the Virgin River.

Follow this pleasant trail with the Virgin River on your right. Within less than a mile, you'll pass the Middle Emerald Pools turnoff on your left, see the wooden fences and barns of the horse corrals on your right, and sight Zion Lodge in the distance across the river. Arriving at a bridge, cross over the Virgin River and walk into the shade of the ancient cottonwood trees in front of Zion Lodge. Here you can browse the gift shops, have lunch, and plan your onward route up the canyon.

TO THE TRAILHEAD

GPS Coordinates: N37º 14.236' W112º 57.439'

From the Zion Canyon Visitor Center, take the Zion Canyon Shuttle to the Court of the Patriarchs stop. In the off-season (November–late March), when the shuttle is not in operation, drive from Canyon Junction (the junction of UT 9 and Zion Canyon Scenic Drive) north on Zion Canyon Scenic Drive for 1.6 miles to the small parking area, on the right side of the road.

WHY DO LIZARDS DO PUSH-UPS?

As you're hiking, you might come across lizards rhythmically raising and lowering their bodies using their front legs, similar to push-ups. Is the lizard working on its biceps, or is it trying to tell you to back off or send some other message? What you are seeing is common among reptiles. They usually exhibit this behavior most frequently in the mornings and evenings. This performance lets

you know that you're in their territory and that they're ready to defend it. Don't expect them to get violent, though—they'll quickly scamper away as you get closer.

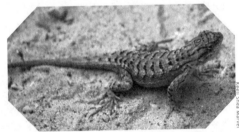

Side-blotched lizard

46 Weeping Rock to Hidden Canyon

Trailhead Location: In Zion Canyon at the Weeping Rock shuttle stop

Trail Use: Walking, hiking

Distance & Configuration: 2.0-mile out-and-back, plus an additional 0.3-mile out-and-back to Weeping Rock

Elevation Range: 4,380' at trailhead to 5,130' at Hidden Canyon entrance

Facilities: Restrooms at Weeping Rock shuttle stop and trailhead

Highlights: At Weeping Rock, seeps in the sandstone cliffs produce hanging gardens. An onward trail leads to a remote side canyon.

DESCRIPTION

Weeping Rock is one of the most popular and easily accessible features in Zion National Park. The landmark is an immense alcove where the lower layer of sandstone has been cut away by erosion, with a seep in the sandstone. As water from the mesa above descends through the upper layers of permeable sandstone, it reaches an impermeable layer and is forced out in seeps, or weeping rocks, on the cliff wall. The constantly trickling water produces an abundance of plant life.

Water sources in a desert environment support up to 500 times more species than the adjacent arid landscape does, so not surprisingly the area surrounding Weeping Rock is marked by

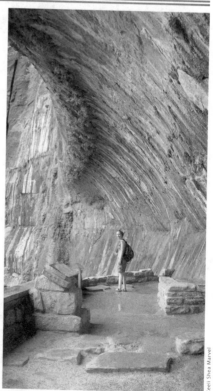

Weeping Rock is a miniature desert oasis.

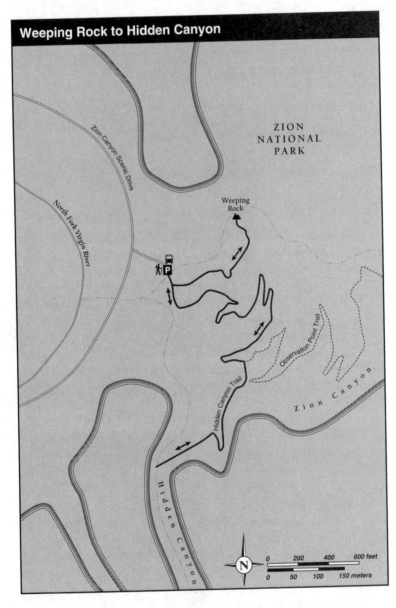

hanging gardens and an assortment of vegetation. Interpretive signs point out trees such as Fremont cottonwood, bigtooth maple, Gambel oak, shrub live oak, velvet ash, and box elder. Smaller shrubs and plants also flourish, and signs identify Oregon grape, hackberry, Palmer's penstemon, three-leaf sumac, and many others. Ferns, lichens, and mosses love the cool shade of the alcove and appear year-round.

The short 0.3-mile round-trip spur trail to Weeping Rock should be part of every visitor's itinerary. It's a fun, fascinating, family-friendly walk along a paved trail, accessible to hikers of virtually all ages, though the steepness of the trail and the broken pavement make it unsuitable for wheelchairs and strollers. Once you've completed the spur, consider the onward trail to Hidden Canyon, described below, or Observation Point, detailed in the next hike profile. Both are well-marked scenic trails; early settlers and American Indians once used these historic routes to access the mesa on foot.

ROUTE

From the south side of the Weeping Rock parking area, cross the bridge and turn left to access Weeping Rock. Once you've returned to the main trail from your Weeping Rock spur, turn left (south) on the trail in the marked direction of Hidden Canyon. You'll ascend against a steep cliff along six long, sweeping switchbacks. Then at 0.6 mile from the trailhead, with the Observation Point Trail taking off to your left, you'll stay to the right in the direction of Hidden Canyon and enter a cluster of tight switchbacks, finally arriving at a rock outcrop capped with a few manzanitas, cacti, piñon pines, shrub live oaks, and ash trees—an interesting array of vegetation. This promontory gives you a great view down and across the canyon. You may decide to make this your stopping point, or you may choose to continue onward and upward in the direction of Hidden Canyon.

The trail continues up along sandstone steps and hugs the canyon wall. A chain placed securely into the wall gives you some added protection. As you work your way to the head of the canyon, the chasm tightens and the trail ascends more than a hundred stairs, taking you into a narrow cleft of the canyon.

At 0.9 mile, the trail crosses the narrow head of the canyon and continues a westward ascent up the canyon's south face. The route is again protected by chains, with steep drop-offs on your right. Moving westward, the path wraps around a fin in a hairpin turn that places you in the mouth of Hidden Canyon. The Hidden Canyon Trail concludes at a large pothole, which may or may not be filled with water depending on the time of year. This pothole marks the entrance to Hidden Canyon and the start of a technical route that requires canyoneering equipment and some solid rock-climbing skills, so for most hikers it's the turnaround point for your descent back to Weeping Rock.

TO THE TRAILHEAD

GPS Coordinates: N37° 16.250' W112° 56.311'

From the Zion Canyon Visitor Center, take the shuttle to the Weeping Rock shuttle stop. In the off-season (November–late March), when the shuttle is not in operation, drive from Canyon Junction (the junction of UT 9 and Zion Canyon Scenic Drive) north on Zion Canyon Scenic Drive for 4.6 miles to the Weeping Rock parking area, on your right.

SEEPS IN SANDSTONE: ANCIENT WATER

Standing in the cool alcove of Weeping Rock with towering cliffs above, you'll see water apparently cascading from a solid sandstone cliff face. You're likely to wonder where the water is coming from. The water you're seeing started as rainfall and snowmelt on the plateau above. The water slowly percolated downward through porous layers of sandstone until it reached an impenetrable layer of rock called the Kayenta Formation; the water had no other way to flow except sideways. From there it found its way out of the cliff in the form of the weeping droplets you see today.

47 Observation Point

Trailhead Location: In Zion Canyon at the Weeping Rock shuttle stop

Trail Use: Walking, hiking

Distance & Configuration: 8.0-mile out-and-back

Elevation Range: 4,380' at trailhead to 6,507' at Observation Point

Facilities: Restrooms at Weeping Rock shuttle stop and parking area

Highlights: Strenuous hike with superb views to the south down Zion Canyon

DESCRIPTION

Three of the park's finest hikes—Weeping Rock, East Rim Trail, and Observation Point—are accessed from the Weeping Rock shuttle stop and trailhead. At this trailhead you're deep in Zion Canyon, the walls rise steeply on all sides, and hanging side canyons finger off in all directions.

Because of the substantial elevation gain from canyon floor to cliff-top plateau—an ascent of more than 2,100 vertical feet—you'll also experience a wide range of ecosystems as you make your climb. From the shaded confines of the canyon floor, with an abundant variety of plant life surrounding

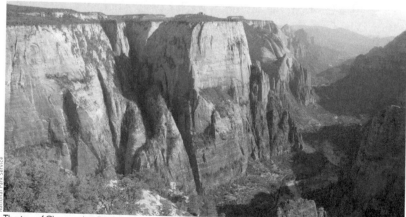

The top of Observation Point

seeps in the sandstone, you'll pass through arid benchlands with cacti and cryptobiotic soil crusts. In the cool shade of Echo Canyon, pockets of ice and snow remain well into spring. But because of seasonal flushing from runoff, vegetation is sparse. Finally, the high-country plateau at the top, which receives more rainfall, lingering snowmelt, and more sun, features a mixed-conifer forest with ponderosa pines and aspens—something you won't see directly below.

Because much of this trail is paved, you'll want to take it easy on the steep descent to avoid too much pounding on your knees. Save those joints for other great hikes in the years to come.

ROUTE

From the south side of the parking area, the paved and well-marked trail takes an immediate fork to the left for a short 0.3-mile round-trip spur up to Weeping Rock (see previous hike), while the longer trail leading to Observation Point continues straight ahead. Don't miss seeing Weeping Rock, but whether you do it as part of this hike to Observation Point or as part of a hike to Hidden Canyon or the East Rim makes little difference.

With the cliffs of The Organ and Angels Landing on your right, the trail veers left and gains its initial ascent on a series of scenic sweeping switchbacks up the east wall of Zion Canyon. Arriving at the junction with the Hidden Canyon Trail, stay to the left as the main trail continues its steep ascent into Echo Canyon. Continuing up the switchbacks, which were blasted out of the canyon wall, you'll quickly have some wonderful views of Weeping Rock and the canyon floor—merely a teaser for the scenery that awaits higher up.

At 2.1 miles from the trailhead, you'll cross the normally dry streambed of Echo Canyon and arrive at a junction. The trail to the right is the East Rim Trail and will lead on a long, looping route to Cable Mountain—for Observation Point, go left. By the time you reach this junction, you've already gained most of your total elevation and covered most of your distance to the top.

After conquering more steep switchbacks, you'll ascend through the White Cliffs formation to arrive at Zion's sandy East Mesa, where the vistas start to open up. For the final mile of the ascent to Observation Point, the trail contours along the lip of the mesa, passes the junction with the East Mesa Trail to the right, and presents some dramatic sights. But the best views are saved for your arrival at Observation Point. As you gaze down Zion Canyon to the south, you'll see several miles of verdant Virgin

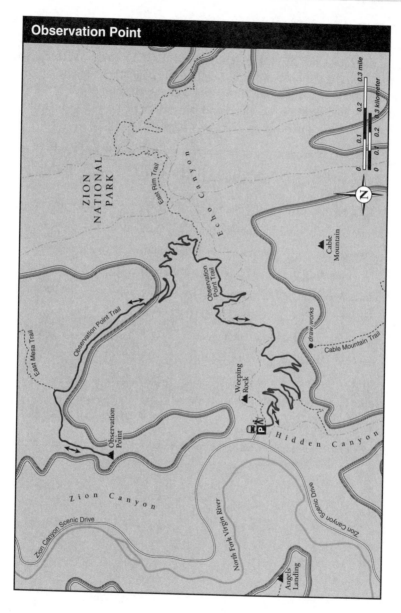

Observation Point

River banks meandering below. The 270-degree panoramas also include spectacular vantage points of Angels Landing and The Organ. It's a well-deserved reward for climbing 2,127 vertical feet. Return the way you came.

TO THE TRAILHEAD

GPS Coordinates: N37º 16.250' W112º 56.311'

From the Zion Canyon Visitor Center, take the shuttle to the Weeping Rock shuttle stop. In the off-season (November–late March), when the shuttle is not in operation, drive from Canyon Junction (the junction of UT 9 and Zion Canyon Scenic Drive) north on Zion Canyon Scenic Drive for 4.6 miles to the Weeping Rock parking area, on your right.

MOUNTAIN LIONS

This elusive, carnivorous mammal can be found throughout the state of Utah. Hunting mainly at night, the mountain lion preys on animals as large as deer as well as smaller animals such as raccoons. Not including the tail, mountain lions are approximately 6 feet long and weigh up to 140 pounds. Once heavily hunted by livestock farmers and ranchers, the big cats are now listed as an endangered species. Though it is rare to see one in person, you may see footprints or scat left behind from one of these amazing creatures.

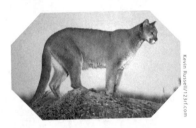

Kevin Russell/123rf.com

48 Riverside Walk

Trailhead Location: At the Temple of Sinawava shuttle stop, at the end of Zion Canyon Scenic Drive

Trail Use: Walking, hiking, wheelchair-accessible

Distance & Configuration: 2.0-mile out-and-back

Elevation Range: 4,438' at trailhead to 4,495' at end of paved trail

Facilities: Water and restrooms at Temple of Sinawava shuttle stop and parking area

Highlights: Entrance to Virgin River Narrows and trailside interpretive signs

DESCRIPTION

The Riverside Walk is the easiest, most accessible, and most inviting hike within Zion National Park. And though the walk is suitable for hikers of all ages and capabilities, the signs at the trailhead provide ample warning of the dangers found in slot canyons and in any outdoor setting. In the case of the Narrows, those dangers can include flash flooding, erupting waterfalls, falling ice, and even avalanches. Rangers do an excellent job of monitoring these hazards, but it's still your responsibility to check advisories and observe warnings to avoid these risks.

The Temple of Sinawava and Riverside Walk are among the park's most beautiful settings, so expect crowds. But even the throng of summer visitors from around the world can do little to detract from this natural splendor.

The Riverside Walk is just a teaser for what lies farther up the canyon. But be forewarned that venturing beyond the paved trail into the Narrows of the Virgin River requires an entirely different level of preparation because the trail quickly gives way to the river. Though the river is rarely more than knee-deep at any point, the rocks on which you'll be walking are like bowling balls, and in the river's current you need rubber-soled shoes, trekking poles or a sturdy staff, and perhaps even a wetsuit in cooler weather.

Hiking the Narrows beyond Riverside Walk is one of the great adventure treks in the Southwest, and it's often rated as one of the best slot-canyon hikes in the world. If it's something you'd like to experience, check first with the visitor center, where rangers will explain the precautions and risks involved, or arrange your trip with one of the experienced commercial outfitters in Springdale.

Riverside Walk

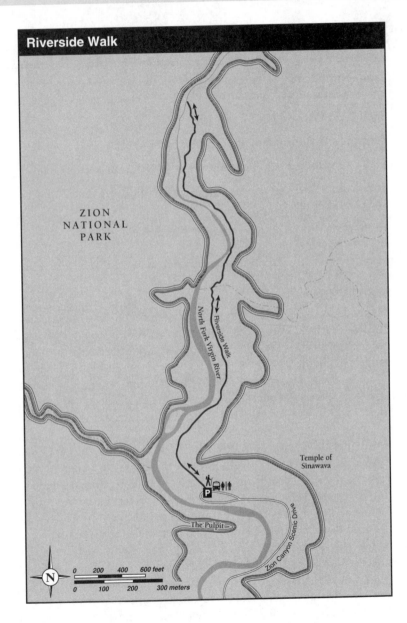

ZION
NATIONAL
PARK

North Fork Virgin River

Riverside Walk

Temple of
Sinawava

P

The Pulpit

Zion Canyon Scenic Drive

0   200   400   600 feet

0   100   200   300 meters

N

ROUTE

Before you embark on your hike, be sure to read the interpretive signs at the trailhead parking area. The signs provide valuable precautionary information about the canyon, especially regarding flash flooding, and also enrich your experience with information about the creation of the Narrows and the natural wonders of the area.

At the trailhead, two imposing towers, the Temple of Sinawava on the right and The Pulpit on the left, flank the mouth of the canyon. However, from your canyon-floor perspective, you can't really see the tops of these towers, just the impressive span of their vertical walls.

As you continue along the paved trail, you'll come across several designated spurs for river access in the first 0.25 mile. These riverside areas are ideal for picnic spots and play.

The paved trail stays to the right of the river. Hikers are treated to hanging gardens and seeping alcoves on the right side of the trail, with riparian woodlands primarily on the left of the path. At 0.6 mile from the trailhead, you arrive at an overhang with benches and guaranteed shade, though shade and cooling temperatures are easy to find in the depths of the Narrows.

The paved trail ends at 1.0 mile as the canyon bends to the northeast. This is the turnaround point for most visitors. If you're willing to get your feet wet, you can venture safely beyond the paved trail for a few hundred yards. To enter the most spectacular reaches of the canyon, though, you'll want to go prepared.

TO THE TRAILHEAD

GPS Coordinates: N37° 17.122' W112° 56.866'
Take the Zion shuttle to the Temple of Sinawava stop, the final stop at the end of Zion Canyon Scenic Drive. By car, from Canyon Junction (the junction of UT 9 and Zion Canyon Scenic Drive), continue north into Zion Canyon for 6.2 miles on Zion Canyon Scenic Drive and park in the Temple of Sinawava parking area.

FLOODING IN THE VIRGIN RIVER

The Virgin River, in its short course of just 170 miles from Navajo Lake to the Colorado River, carries with it 100 million tons of debris, silt, and particulates every year. The vast majority of that occurs in just 15–20 days of flooding each year.

49 Taylor Creek

Trailhead Location: On the east side of Kolob Canyons Road, 1.9 miles east of the Kolob Canyons Visitor Center

Trail Use: Walking, hiking

Distance & Configuration: 5.0-mile out-and-back

Elevation Range: 5,444' at Taylor Creek near trailhead to 5,894' at Double Arch Alcove

Facilities: None

Highlights: Two historic cabins, towering sandstone cliffs, a perennial spring-fed creek, and Double Arch Alcove

DESCRIPTION

Note: Extreme weather conditions can cause flash flooding in this section of Zion National Park.

Zion's Kolob Canyons section is often referred to as a park within a park. Kolob Canyons was once a national monument, separate from Zion National Park, and it has its own visitor center accessed from I-15, nearly an hour away from Zion Canyon and the park's main attractions.

Kolob Canyons consists of a series of deep and narrow finger canyons at the western edge of the Colorado Plateau. The 5-mile scenic drive ends at a high viewpoint. But the spectacular scenery of Kolob Canyons is best seen on foot, as numerous trails ascend into the remote upper reaches of the canyons along streambeds and with towering canyon walls overhead.

Taylor Creek is the ideal initiation into the scenic wonders of Kolob Canyons. The trail winds through a designated wilderness area and passes two early-20th-century cabins before arriving at Double Arch Alcove, a large grotto with a sandstone arch suspended high overhead.

The Taylor Creek Trail combines many of Zion's signature features in a short distance: sheer cliffs, deeply incised streams, diverse vegetation, natural springs, and unusual geologic formations—all of which can be enjoyed without the crowds found in Zion Canyon.

The deep woods along Taylor Creek invite songbirds, deer, and many small mammals, including foxes and skunks. In summer you'll also encounter biting flies, which seem to be undisturbed by insect repellent.

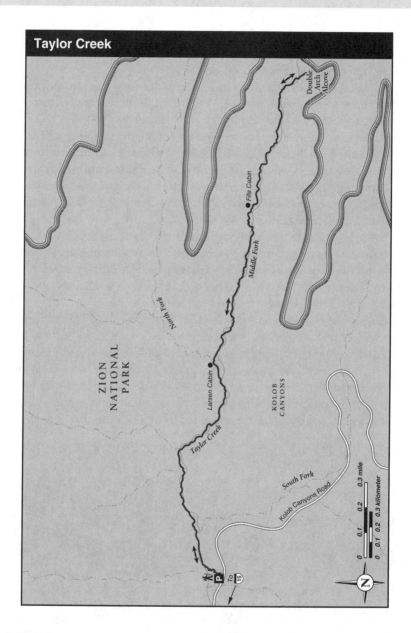

Taylor Creek

ROUTE

From the trailhead parking area on Kolob Canyons Road, the trail quickly descends 350 feet along a stairway, arriving at a creek that invites play. The creek makes for an appealing stop, even though you're just a few minutes into the hike. The banks and slopes lining the creek bear evidence of erosion on a regular basis due to flash flooding.

At the TAYLOR CREEK TRAIL sign, the path follows the stream, crossing continually from bank to bank. You'll have no fewer than 30 stream crossings as you ascend the canyon, but it's doubtful that your feet will ever get wet because the water is shallow—never more than a couple inches deep.

Continuing up the creek, you'll pass bigtooth maples, noble firs, cottonwoods, tamarisks, and willows. At 0.9 mile, you come to an alcove that provides some welcome shade in the heat of summer. Continuing on for another 0.2 mile, you'll arrive at the Larsen cabin, dating to the 1930s, with interpretive signs that detail its history.

In less than a mile, and at about 2.1 miles from the trailhead, you arrive at the second cabin, the Fife cabin, which was the mountain home of sheep ranchers more than 80 years ago. After passing the Fife cabin, the trail turns into the stream and vice versa, although the water is so shallow and the rocks so abundant that crossings are fun and feet stay dry.

Despite the fact that you're on one of the less-traveled routes in the depth of a wooded canyon, the trail is well defined, well marked, and easy to follow. After veering to the right, you arrive at Double Arch Alcove, 2.5 miles from the trailhead. The moss-covered grotto is wet with seeps from the Navajo Sandstone, and the moisture creates a microhabitat with bigtooth maples, ferns, and conifers. This alcove is the source of most of the water in the stream, although the stream is also fed by other springs in the area. To

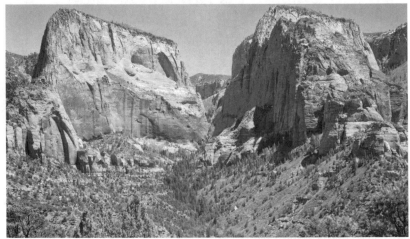

Kolob Canyons

protect the wildflowers and to prevent further erosion in the canyon, stay on the trail and don't venture up the canyon beyond the alcove. Enjoy the niche's natural air-conditioning and wonderful acoustics before returning the way you came.

TO THE TRAILHEAD
GPS Coordinates: N37° 27.712' W113° 11.967'
From the Kolob Canyons Visitor Center, continue eastward into the park on Kolob Canyons Road for 1.9 miles. The Taylor Canyon Trailhead and parking area are on the left.

INVASIVE SPECIES

Not all the plants found in national parks are native species or even desirable—some are invasive and cause havoc to the natural ecosystem. One such invasive plant is the tamarisk, also known as saltcedar. Identified by its feathery leaves and pink flowers, it was originally introduced from Eurasia as an ornamental shrub. Its foliage can grow up to 25 feet high and blocks light and space from other plants. It deposits salt on the ground, making other vegetation unable to grow. Mainly found along streams and near water sources, this plant blocks water access for many animals, and tamarisk is not edible for many of the native wildlife. Scientists are currently trying to eradicate this plant by introducing tamarisk leaf beetles, as well as by using prescribed burns, and have found some success. Despite the efforts, tamarisk is plentiful and is not going away anytime soon.

50 Cable Mountain Trail

Trailhead Location: On the park's eastern boundary near Zion Ponderosa Ranch

Trail Use: Walking, hiking

Distance & Configuration: 7.4-mile out-and-back

Elevation Range: 6,452' at trailhead to 6,700' on the crest of the trail on Cable Mountain

Facilities: None

Highlights: A glimpse into the history of logging in the area and spectacular vistas into Zion Canyon from a lofty viewpoint

DESCRIPTION

Cable Mountain is barely recognizable from the depths of Zion Canyon. It's just another spot along the rim and hardly worth comparing to some of Zion's magnificent thrones or cathedrals. But Cable Mountain's historical significance, coupled with the view you'll get into Zion Canyon, make this hike an incomparable experience.

When early settlers began looking for sources of timber to supply Zion Canyon, Cable Mountain was a natural choice, with an abundant forest of Douglas-firs and pines. The only problem was that it was 2,000 feet straight above the canyon floor, which meant that several days of travel by wagon were required to get the timber off the mountain and into Zion Canyon. Lumbermen devised an inventive solution to move the timber to the canyon floor, shaving days off the trip, and you'll enjoy seeing the remains of their creativity.

The Cable Mountain trailhead is on the park's eastern boundary, so you'll need to exit the park to the east on UT 9. If you're arriving in Zion after visiting Bryce Canyon, you may want to consider doing this hike before entering the park to avoid backtracking.

Because much of the Cable Mountain trail was used as a wagon road in the early 20th century, the path is wide and easy to follow, with signs at all trail junctions. It's not unusual to spend an hour or more on the trail and never see another hiker. Instead, you'll have expansive views across the plateau in all directions before arriving at the rim, where you'll enjoy breathtaking views down into the canyon.

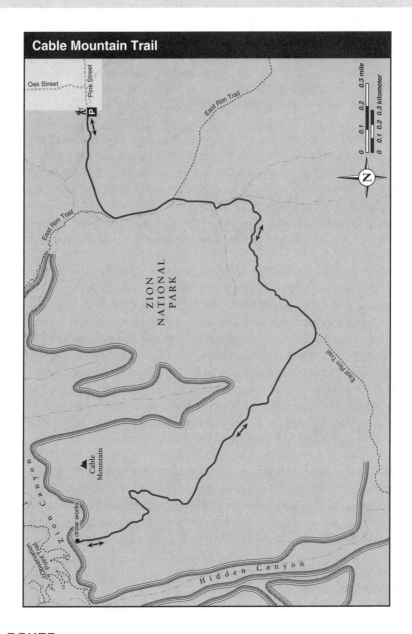

Cable Mountain Trail

ROUTE

From the trailhead parking area, the trail heads west on a level course across a ponderosa-and-sage plateau. At 0.5 mile, you arrive at a junction with a north–south trail—take the route to the left for Cable Mountain.

Here the trail begins to gently ascend a wide draw to the south, with outcrops of red rock on the left. At 0.3 mile from the first junction, you arrive at a second junction with Stave Springs, where the original sawmill on Cable Mountain was located, marked on the left—instead, stay to the right, with the sign indicating Cable Mountain 3.0 miles down the trail to the west.

From this junction the trail ascends the right side of the draw, and the grade steepens a bit. Even though you're on a sparsely wooded plateau, you have good views in all directions, including views of the Paunsaugunt Plateau to the east, the location of Bryce Canyon. For early settlers, the plateau you're traversing would have been favorable grazing land with more moisture than other regions to the east. On this plateau, the trail is wreathed with Indian paintbrushes and arrowleaf balsamroots, among other wildflowers.

At 1.1 miles from the previous trail junction, near the crest of this wide and open plateau, you arrive at a fork in the road, with Deertrap Mountain to the left and Cable Mountain to the right. Bear right.

Once you're past this intersection, the trail stays fairly level, with only slight undulations before coming to two large trees, one on each side of the trail; here the descent to the rim of Cable Mountain begins. Less than a mile after departing the junction, you'll have your first views of Zion Canyon. Soon the trail begins a steep descent along rubbly surface. At this point on the path, you'll have distant views of the draw works to the right.

Finally, at 3.7 miles from the trailhead and after hooking to the northwest, the trail arrives at the end of the promontory, where the sturdy and recently restored draw works are planted firmly on the rim. As with other backcountry overviews in Zion, no fence protects you from the 2,000-foot plunge to the canyon floor. You'll want to get as close as possible for the best views into the canyon and to Observation Point on the promontory to the north, but use extra caution. Nearby trees offer a shady spot for a lunch or snack before returning to the trailhead the way you came.

TO THE TRAILHEAD

GPS Coordinates: N37° 16.063' W12° 53.969'

From Zion National Park's east entrance station, drive east on UT 9 for 2.4 miles to North Fork Road. Turn left (north) onto North Fork Road and continue for 5.3 miles to the entrance of Zion Ponderosa Ranch Resort, on the left. Turn left onto Twin Knolls Road and continue for 1.2 miles, and then turn left on Buck Road. At the first junction, bear right and continue for 0.6 mile to a Y in the road. Bear left onto West Pine Street and continue for 0.5 mile to the gate marking the park boundary. With a high-clearance vehicle, you can make the steep descent and enter through the gate into the small parking area. Otherwise, park in one of the small roadside pads east of the gate, but don't block the narrow dirt road. Be sure to close the gate behind you to keep livestock from wandering into the park.

THE CABLE MOUNTAIN DRAW WORKS

In 1901, David Flannigan built a cableway, or a draw works, on the rim of Cable Mountain high above Zion Canyon to quickly move lumber from the East Rim to the floor of Zion Canyon. The 2,000-foot cable descent allowed him to lower lumber in 2 minutes, saving many days of travel by wagon over rough roads. From 1904 to 1907, Flannigan ran a steam-powered sawmill at Stave Springs, which you'll pass near the Cable Mountain Trail. The cable lowered the lumber and shingles used in the building of the original Zion Lodge and cabins. The draw works burned in 1911 after being struck by

lightning, and a second fire destroyed the rebuilt frame in the early 1920s. Dwindling timber supplies on the East Rim eventually forced the closure of the sawmill and eliminated the need for the draw works, which ceased operation in 1930.

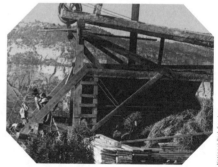

National Park Service

NATIONAL PARK CONTACT INFORMATION

Arches National Park
435-719-2299
435-719-2100
nps.gov/arch

Bryce Canyon National Park
435-834-5322
nps.gov/brca

Canyonlands National Park
Island in the Sky: 435-259-4712
The Needles: 435-259-4711
The Maze: 435-259-2652
nps.gov/cany

Capitol Reef National Park
435-425-3791, ext. 4111
nps.gov/care

Zion National Park
435-772-3256
nps.gov/zion

INDEX

About the Author

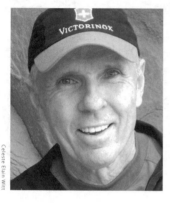

Celeste Elain Witt

Greg Witt has lived the adventures he writes about and shares with audiences around the world. His journeys have taken him to every corner of the globe. He has guided mountaineering expeditions in the Alps and Andes and paddled wild rivers in the Americas. He has dropped teams of adventurers into golden slot canyons; trudged through deep jungles in Africa, Central America, and Asia; and guided archeological expeditions across the parched Arabian Peninsula. His passion for adventure has always focused on sharing his experience with others.

After earning degrees from the University of California and Brigham Young University, Greg had an early career in human-resources management. However, he prefers high adventure to the high-rise, so decades ago he traded his wingtips for hiking boots and has never looked back.

Greg is the founder and chief adventure officer of Alpenwild, the leading outfitter of hiking and trekking trips in the Alps. Some weeks he hikes more miles than he drives, which means that he wears out his boots faster than he wears out his tires. He has crossed the Grand Canyon on foot many times, climbed Colorado's three highest peaks in three days, and in a recent summer in the Swiss Alps hiked more than 700 miles and gained nearly 100,000 vertical feet of elevation—the equivalent of climbing Everest nine times.

As a guidebook writer, Greg leads readers on the most breathtaking hikes and exciting outdoor adventures on the globe. He loves to discuss the geology, history, archaeology, weather patterns, culture, flora, and fauna of his favorite locales. His other books include *60 Hikes Within 60 Miles: Salt Lake City* (Menasha Ridge Press) and *Ultimate Adventures: A Rough Guide to Adventure Travel* (Rough Guides). He is the US editor of *Off the Tourist Trail: 1,000 Unexpected Travel Alternatives* (DK Eyewitness Travel) and a contributing editor of *Make the Most of Your Time on Earth: A Rough Guide to the World* (Rough Guides).

Greg's research and exploration continue to uncover the unknown, as well as surprising adventures just waiting to be experienced. If you join him, you can be guaranteed a phenomenal adventure peppered with the unexpected.